Today's bookshelves contain many volumes which claim to have discovered the answer to back problems. *Do this exercise* or *follow that program* and your back pain will disappear and be no more.

And yet the incidence of back problems in this country is increasing at an alarming rate. Doctors are saying "if this were a virus, we'd call it an epidemic!" How can this be? If the solution is at hand, why is the problem growing so fast? Could it be that there are other, more subtle reasons for back pains than what are being proposed?

Back Talk makes no such exaggerated claims as to having *the solution* to back pain. The author's own experience and research indicates that there are a variety of solutions. What may be effective for one may not be for another.

This book presents an overview of back problems—what they may be, how they work and what may be done for them. More importantly, it examines closely the interaction between back pain and the individual's physical and emotional state. For it is only through knowledge and understanding that we may start to combat this complex malady.

THROUGH KNOWLEDGE COMES UNDERSTANDING, WITH UNDERSTANDING, HEALTH.

Low back pain is one of the most common conditions seen by the practitioner and results in an annual loss of 1,400 work days per 1,000 workers in the United States.
Thomas P. Sculco, MD
The Manuscript of Rheumatology and Outpatient Orthopedic Disorders

Pain in the neck and/or back...is one of man's most common afflictions...Because the pathophysiology of most such pain is poorly understood, the physician often encounters patients for whom he can neither make a certain diagnosis nor prescribe rational therapy.

Jerome B. Posner, MD
Professor of Neurology
Cornell University Medical College
Cecil Textbook of Medicine

....most acute low back pain is diagnostically nonspecific...

Brendon M. Reilly, MD
Practical Strategies In Outpatient Medicine

BACK TALK

J. Robert DuBois

Bannister Publications

Copyright ©1987 Bannister Publications

Library of Congress Catalog Card Number 87-72087

ISBN **0-916885-04-6** (soft cover)
ISBN **0-916885-05-4** (hard cover)

A *Bannister Book*

First edition
First printing October, 1987

Printed in the United States of America

Atlas Art by Rebecca Slattery

To my wife, Karen, for all these years of patience, understanding, and love.

In my experience 85% of back pains are not specifically diagnosed...No one knows what it is.

> **Dr. Alf Nachelson**
> Orthopedic surgeon and
> Leading authority on back pain
> Sweden
> (from an inverview on ABC Nightly News, Sept. 9, 1985)

TABLE OF CONTENTS

ILLUSTRATIONS

Acknowledgements

Few projects of this type are completed without the help of others. Such is certainly the case with this book. At the top of the list are my parents, Jack and Thelma, and my wife, Karen, without whose nurturing and support I would not be writing this. Over the many years they have extended an understanding which has occasionally surpassed all limits of expectation.

My children, Rob, Diane and Sheri, have many times had to do without the catching partner or hiking companion they would have liked their father to be, and yet they never complained. Instead, they offered care and encouragement.

A special thanks to Charles Spaulding, DC for the help with my back I had not found elsewhere. He is the man who got me back up and around and allows me to stay there. And it is certainly easier to work at a typewriter than having to scratch out material in longhand in bed.

And speaking of writing, I want to make a special mention of Joseph W. Zarzynski and his lovely young bride, Pat Meaney. *Zarr* and I struggled through the *first book syndrome* a few years ago and together learned a lot about the wonderful and wacky world of books.

The list of supportive friends is long, but needs to include Erik and Janet Hansen who provided the inspira-

Acknowledgements

tion for the title of this book, Ray and Karen Manley, Jerry Williams, Al Blanche and Larry and Emma Jeffers who helped distribute questionaires for the survey and provided the occasional verbal kick-in-the-butt to keep me writing. Jack Hughes, for providing the great belly laugh and break in the tedium of proofreading with his *typo* of "the insecure king and his band of lock washers," and Bill Milliken, from whom I am still learning the value of patience. One step at a time and one word at a time, right Bill?

For helping with the research for this book, I need to mention Rory Gillespie for the loan of all his medical books, Shirley Trudell, LPN of Yankee Medical for her courteous assistance, and Rowland Hazard, MD, Steven Kalisch, PhD and Ken Yates, of the New England Back Center, for their refreshing attitudes and generous time.

And last but certainly not least, I want to thank the Harmony House Players for helping others see the lighter side of life and advocating the value of a good sense of humor, and acknowledge Wolfgang Erik Schmuhl and all those unnamed Army buddies who helped carry my field pack all those many years ago. It may have seemed like a small thing to you guys, but it made all the difference to me in being able to finish that damnable hike that day my back was out.

JRD

Foreword

When anyone mentions a bad back the image which often comes to mind is something akin to the Rob Petri routine on the Dick Van Dyke Show. A man bends over to pick an item up off the floor, develops a strange look on his face, and starts walking around in an "L" position. We can tell its supposed to hurt by the grimace of pain on his face and the fact that he says it does. A few wise cracks are than exchanged by the onlookers such as *can't be a pretzel, its too big,* or *we could put a doily on his back and have a new end table,* or *the next time I lose a contact lens I'll give you a call.* And all this is funny, right? You bet Aunt Fanny's falsies it is. Unless it happens to you. Then...but more about that, later.

One of the interesting elements of these celluloid situations is the cure. It usually consists of a friend or associate placing his hands on the sufferer's shoulders, his knee in the small of the sore back, and pulling sharply upwards. We then hear someone stepping on walnuts and the former patient stands upright, smiles, and pronounces himself cured. And the show goes on...long live the show.

While I have heard of such miraculous recoveries actually taking place at times, it has never been my good fortune to see one personally. My own experience dictates that when such an injury has taken place it usually takes some time to heal properly. Certain treatments are available which may shorten that time and some items may make that time more bearable, but injuries must heal to be well.

In case you question the use of the word *injury* in such a situation, rest assured that is in fact the case. While it may not be as dramatic as a baseball to the head or an arrow in the shoulder, it is an injury nonetheless. The causes and types of these injuries are addressed later in the book, along with methods of treatment and prevention, so I will not go into detail here. It will be sufficient at this point to state that most back problems are originally the result of injury. Where back injuries become such a major problem, however, is in the complexity of the back itself.

If you break an arm or sprain an ankle, you are usually able to wear a cast or use crutches for a period of time to avoid usage of the afflicted area while it heals. Backs are not quite so simple. As we will see later, backs are a delicate balancing mechanism which don't require much to throw them out of whack. While a strong back may be able to lift tremendous weights when prepared, a sudden or jerky movement may well result in a pulling of one of the many muscles or ligaments on one side of the back. Because of the balancing role the back plays for most of the body, other muscles may be called into action to counter-balance or protect the weakened area. These "defender of the down-trodden" muscles might well be forced into service for which they are not trained and end up in spasm or cramping.

Once things have reached this point the rest of the process is as easy as rolling downhill in a garbage can. The resultant muscle contractions and inflamation can contort the spine, compress discs, squeeze nerves to radiate pain into other parts of the body (the sciatic is a common target for this) and generally wreak havoc with most things you hold near and dear. All you know is that you hurt like hell and can't move very well. Your back is now *out*.

If all of this sounds complicated (it does) and a little frightening (that, too), it is nevertheless quite common. According to recent statistics some eighty million people in the United States suffer from one back problem or another during their lives. Add to this the new finding that over the last decade or so the incidence of back problems has increased several times faster than the population growth, that bad backs are already the leading cause of lost work time in this country, and we can easily see how severe this issue has become.

Now that we have covered most of the gloom and doom, however, lets take an even closer look at the good news.

In most cases back problems are not permanent. The time spent in bed during an "attack" may seen like an eternity, but it really isn't. And there are things you can do to not only shorten the duration and lessen the severity of an episode, but in fact maybe prevent its recurrence. We can all be more in control of our own lives and make them a better experience.

During the course of this book we will be looking at the *whats, whys* and *hows* of bad backs and examining our relationships with them. We will be hearing from medical doctors, chiropractors, osteopaths and the guy down the street. There will be plenty of facts and figures for the most statistically minded of individuals and maybe even a photograph or two of a pretty girl for the more esthetically oriented. And interspersed throughout will be an occasional glimpse of humor. Humor? There's nothing funny about a bad back, is there? Maybe a bit of my personal background would be appropriate here.

For over 20 years I spent anywhere from several days to several weeks a year laid up with a bad back. I experienced fully the pain and depression these bouts can generate. Each time I felt as if my life had fallen completely apart and wondered if I would ever lead a normal life again. And then one day during a period of recuperation I thought about an experience I'd had during a previous episode which was almost humorous. I say almost humorous because nothing seemed very funny at the time. I did feel a little better, however, just thinking about the occurence.

And at that stage of the game anything helped. The more I looked, the more humor I found and the better I felt. Not physically, at first, but emotionally, anyway. That gave me the incentive to explore further, so I started jotting down the experiences which came to mind, both as a therapy and for future reference. All of these notes had to be written in longhand on whatever paper was available at the time because I was unable to sit up at a typewriter. Or anywhere else, for that matter.

After two or three years of such idle scribbling and passing of time I realized that what was helping me might just help others in the same boat. So I started assembling the random bits of paper I had accumulated over the years and began doing some serious research on back pain.

What I found was most interesting and very helpful, and eventually became the book you are now reading. (At the time of this writing I have been back on my feet for over four years and feeling great.) I hope the information benefits you as much as it has me.

If you are reading this in bed with a heating pad and a bottle of aspirin, so much the better. It is for just such times that this book was written. So read on, enjoy, and indulge yourself an occasional chuckle at my expense.

I wish you a speedy recovery and a healthy rest of your life.

Chapter 1

THE BACK

To say the human body is a complex machine is to say that Enrico Caruso was a good singer. Andy Williams is a good singer. Johnny Cash, to some, is a good singer. Enrico Caruso was one of the outstanding voices of all time. A race car is a complex machine. The space shuttle is a complex machine. The human body is an interrelated network of componants which exceeds imagination. It consists of bones, muscles, ligaments, tendons, blood, nerves, electrical impulses, senses, organs and a bunch of other things I can't begin to understand completely. Nor can anyone else for that matter. The more the human body is studied the more complex the interworkings of the individual componants are made apparent. I personally don't know how or why human anatomy was developed or who or what developed it, but I would strongly recommend further study to all of us. The more we can learn about ourselves the more fully will we appreciate this machine each of us inhabits which enables us to see, hear, feel, smell, taste, sing, think, move about, remember, procreate and nurture our young. A mechanism which is generally able to repair its own breakdowns, provided only a modicum of maintenance by its owner.

This, however, is neither a lecture on theology nor a discourse on anatomy. It is simply a layman's guide to low back pain, so I will get back to the subject at hand.

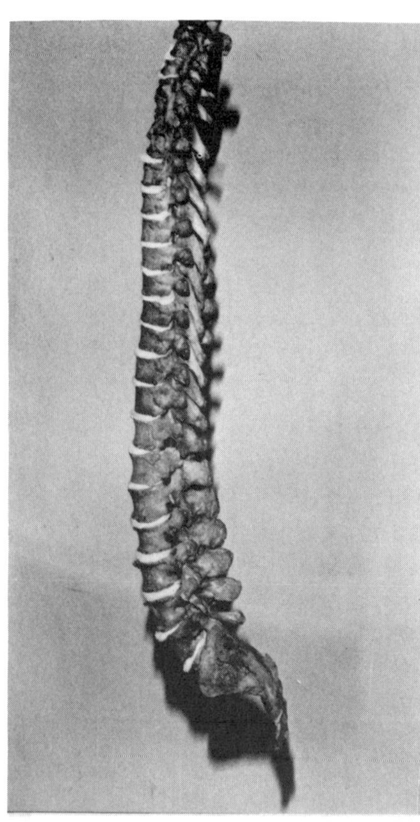

A human spine as viewed from the side. The vertebral stack (from top to bottom) consists of the Cervical Spine, C1--C7 (neck), the Thoracic or Dorsal Spine, T1--T12 (mid-back), and the Lumbar Spine, L1--L5). The large bone at the bottom is the Sacrum, with the Coccyx (tailbone) at the lower tip. (Because of the difficulty encountered in posing a spine, this specimen does not reflect the natural inward curve in the Lumbar Spine region which would be found in a healthy backbone.)

The back, or more specifically, the spine, is the support column or standard bearer for the bulk of the body. It is analogous to the foundation of a building, without which the structure would collapse.

The spine consists of 24 movable bones (vertebrae) stacked on top of each other and separated by 23 discs. The discs act as shock absorbers, reducing friction between the vertebrae and allowing freedom of movement of the spine.

Through this column of bones run the three different parts of the nervous system, starting in the brain and traveling down and through the spine to service every living tissue in the body. These consist of the Central Nervous System which is the spinal cord (encased in the center of the spinal vertebrae for protection), the Autonomic Nervous System (or *involuntary nervous system* which governs automatic body functions such as heartbeat, digestion and circulation) and the Peripheral Nervous System which connects the central nervous system with the various tissues of the body.

It is through this network of interdependent and interrelated segments of the nervous system that pain and function messages travel. Injuries to the spine from accident, stress, tension or any other factor which causes minor displacement or derangement of the vertebrae can cause irritation to spinal nerve roots which, in turn, may cause malfunctions elsewhere in the body. It is for this reason that practitioners of chiropractic pay such attention to the alignment of the spine. Only through proper alignment of this bony conduit can the nervous system serve its proper purpose and keep the body functioning as intended.

Now add to all this the complicated musculature system of the back. These muscles have to work not only in lifting, bending, turning, twisting and all other movements of the body, they have to help support and maintain alignment of the support system we have just discussed. In addition, they have to work in harmony with their opposite members on the other side of the body. A strained muscle in the back will often require overexertion in the way of compensation by another muscle, thereby aggravating the existing condition. It is during such times that sciatic scoliosis (leaning) may occur. As discussed in the chapter on leaning, sciatic scoliosis is usually not life threatening, but is certainly an indication that something is wrong.

Interestingly enough, this situation will usually clear itself up in time. As Dr. Reilly puts it in *Practical Strategies in Outpatient Medicine,* "most acute simple mechanical back pain resolves spontaniously..." this is not to say that back pain should be ignored. I'm not sure it can be ignored for that matter, it demands too much attention. But after

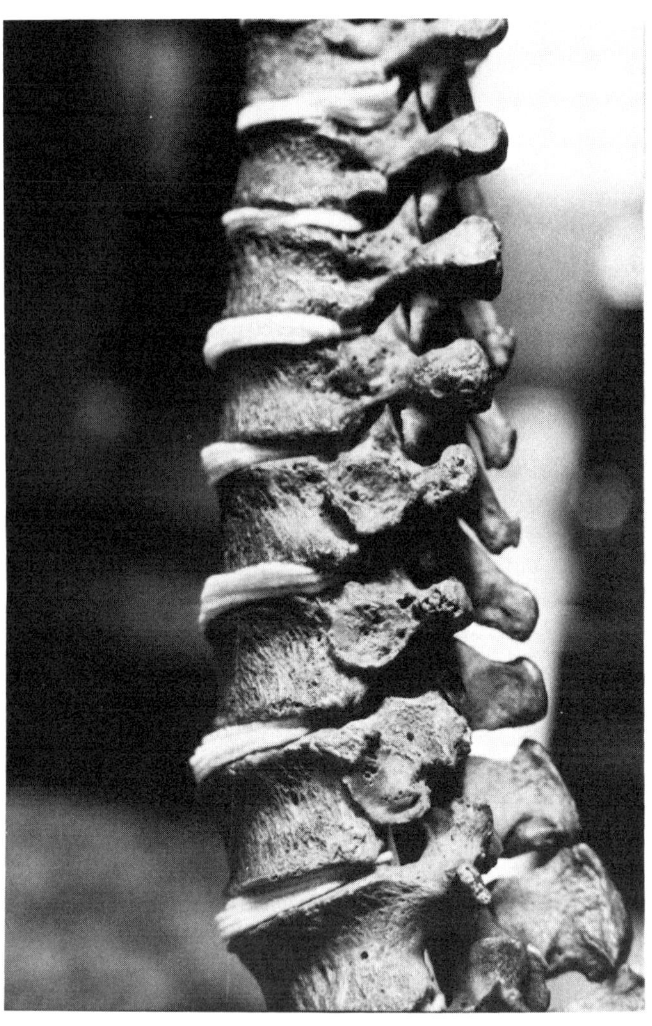

A close-up shot of the lower Dorsal and Upper Lumbar area of the same spine. The felt inserts between the vertebrae represent what would be the discs in a living spine. Note the irregular surface of the bodies of the vertebrae: This indicates the existance of osteoporosis which is often found in the elderly, especially in women.

thorough examination by a physician and elimination of any specific, physiological causes, it often becomes a matter of patience until the matter clears up.

There are methods, however, whereby that healing process may be greatly accelerated and the time required for recovery reduced dramatically. These are rest, mild exercise, relaxation, chiropractic treatment and awareness. Since they are all covered in detail elsewhere, I will touch upon them only lightly here.

Rest is conducive to healing. If your body is fatigued and overextended it cannot focus on the area to be repaired. Mild exercise means just that, *mild* exercise to limber and loosen tight muscles. Relaxation goes hand-in-hand with the above and is the intentional letting-go of muscles which are being clenched to protect against the actual or anticipated pain. These are generally accepted methods of dealing with injury, especially in cases of simple mechanical back pain. The forth method, chiropractic treatment, may not be as universally accepted, but in my experience has been invaluable. I suffered from prolonged episodes of low back pain for over 20 years until my wife finally convinced me to see a chiropractor. I was desperate enough to *try anything,* and I'm glad I did. (See Chapter 8: What About Chiropractic?)

Awareness is...well, lets not jump the gun. We'll get to that in due time.

Chronic back pain affects people's moods, relationships, their work lives, and physically speaking, their whole bodies, because its not just the back that gets out of shape.
Rowland Hazard, MD
Medical Director
New England Back Center

Chapter 2

CAUSES OF BACK PAIN

"In my experience 85% of back pains are not specifically diagnosed...no one knows what it is." (Dr. Alf Nachelson, orthopedic surgeon and leading authority on back pain, from ABC Nightly News, September 9, 1985.) To start a chapter which even pretends to explain what back pain is with Dr. Nachelson's statement would seem to be misleading at least, and perhaps an exercise in futility at worst. However there it is. My own experience, as mentioned elsewhere in this book, was five different diagnoses from as many practitioners before my problem was discovered and effectively treated. Does this suggest, then, that you should just forget trying to get help and go through life suffering stoically? Not at all. But it does certainly suggest a second or perhaps even third opinion before embarking on an involved and perhaps expensive treatment program. And, in my opinion, it suggests looking at various options available to you, not just cheerfully jumping up on the operating table for the first surgeon who waves a knife in front of you, if such should be the case. There are certainly situations where surgery would seem to be the answer, but there have also been many instances in which surgery was advised, which were resolved with less dramatic measures.

In any event it is not my job to tell you what the source of your pain is or what the best treatment would be. My job right now is simply to list some of the major sources of back pain. And here they are.

1. CHRONIC TRAUMA — as caused by poor posture, for example, and which develops over a period of time. The spine of humans contains four natural curves designed to properly support the weight of the body in an erect position. When these natural curves are modified or amended due to poor posture, the ligaments, tendons and muscles are forced to work in an unnatural fashion and abnormal stresses and strains may occur.

2. SUDDEN TRAUMA — unlike chronic trauma which develops slowly, sudden trauma is just what the name implies. If you are body-tackled by a defensive lineman and find you have trouble moving, you have just experienced sudden trauma. It doesn't need to be nearly as dramatic as this, however. It can result from a sudden twisting or lifting movement, but the effect is the same — you have experienced an immediate and painful injury.

3. SLIPPED DISC — a few years ago one of the most popular diagnosis for back problems. A disc is the circular little *shock absorber* located between the vertebrae which allows for movement of the spine. If a disc is damaged by either sudden or chronic trauma it may distend or rupture. This, then, in effect, *loses the seal* for which the disc was designed and a complete breakdown of the intervertebral joint takes place. The shock absorbing function of the disc is then lost, the spine alters its balance and the surrounding muscles and ligaments have to overcompensate to take up the load. A couple of the pains which may result from this are *lumbago,* in which the muscles of the back suddenly completely lock up for a period of time (and may just as suddenly unlock), and *sciatica,* in which the distension of the disc material will press on the spinal cord or nerve roots branching out from it and cause the old familiar pain shooting down the back of one or both legs.

4. ARTHRITIS — another popular diagnosis for back

pain, although the actual occurance may not be quite as common as the diagnosis. Arthritis is broken down into two types — *osteoarthritis,* a mechanical wearing process, and *rheumatoid arthritis,* a disease.

Osteoarthritis is by far the most common type of arthritis. It can affect the entire spine, but usually involves the areas which have the most movement. Just as any hinge or motion-involved mechanical part will wear down after long periods of use, so do the joints of the spine start to wear out with age or prolonged abuse. Interestingly enough, the development of osteoarthritis may lead to a natural fusion of the vertebrae above and below the effected disc joint. This can then lead to a lessening of the pain since no further motion can take place at that joint.

Rheumatoid Arthritis is a less common but more serious form of arthritis. As a disease, it usually starts in the large joints of the body and spreads to other joints, involving the spine usually in the later stages. One of the main problems with rheumatoid arthritis is that it creates a thinning of the density of the bone and causes osteoporosis, which we have all heard so much about on television commercials lately. Fortunately it is a relatively rare disease and is probably not the reason you are reading this book.

5. THE AGING PROCESS — One of the personal questions I have had concerning life is: why do we age? And how? In doing research for this book I was relieved (I suppose) to discover that no one else seems to know the answer either. Suffice it to say that we *do* age, and in so doing are subject to certain changes in our bodies. One of these is that we lose some of the water content of our body's tissues. This is of some importance when discussing the spine as it tends to start aging (and drying) sooner than other parts of the body. As the discs in the spine start to lose their water content they start shrinking, leading to a reduction in the length of the spine and subsequently a reduction in overall height. As this takes place, again, the supportive ligaments are forced to take up the slack and chronic strain begins.

No discussion of the spine and aging would be complete without going into osteoporosis, as mentioned above. Osteoporosis is also caused by other than rhumatoid arthritis. It can come about by simple aging, as well as be a byproduct of the hormone imbalance of women who have gone through the menopause. Interestingly enough, for postmenopausal osteoporosis and especially for senile osteoporosis (due to aging), bed rest is not very effective. Unlike trauma, where there is an injury which needs to heal, this is a condition which needs muscle support to compensate for the weakening bones of the spine. Bed rest only helps further deteriorate those muscles upon which you are so dependent. If it is any consolation, most of us will develop senile osteoporosis to one degree or another. Provided we live long enough, that is.

6. PREGNANCY — Although far from my field of experience, I understand many women experience back pain during, and sometimes after, pregnancy. The reason for this would seem to be self explanatory — a shift in body alignment, redistribution of body weight and increase of weight supported, all of which puts greater strain on the muscles and ligaments of the back. Much of this discomfort may be alleviated by a proper exercise program to strengthen the back. These exercises should take place before, during and after the pregnancy. Once again, consult with your doctor or health practitioner to determine what type of program is best for you. (See: For Women Only)

7. PSYCHOLOGICAL — Now we are into one of my favorite areas. Chances are good you have had at least one doctor or, better yet, friend or relative, tell you your problem is all in your mind, its psychosomatic. Lets talk about this a bit.

Traditionally, when a doctor is unable to find a specific, clinical problem causing the pain, he or she will tell you there is nothing wrong with your back. And we really can't blame them. Pain is a difficult element to measure and different people have varying amounts of pain tollerance. Plus the fact we have all seen or heard about the neck brace that is worn for severe whiplash, until the day after the court appearance, anyway, at which time a miraculous and speedy healing process takes place. Sure there is fraud in our society. The problem is, for every fraudulant case that takes place, there are many more real cases of severe and debilitating injury. Again, the problem — you can see a broken leg or a bullet hole, but a sprained muscle or pulled ligament is obvious only to the individual wearing it. So now we have a situation of someone claiming to be in pain with no apparent cause. If you were the doctor what would you do? Probably one of two or three things. You could refer them on to a specialist in hopes of something specific being discovered or you could treat them with a placebo so at least the patient would think they are being treated. Or you could tell that patient to go home, that there is nothing wrong with them, that it is all in their mind.

I know a woman who complained of chronic back pain for years. Nothing severe, just a constant nagging ache. After consulting several physicians and being told by all that nothing was physiologically wrong with her, she began to wonder. Finally a new doctor discovered her uterus was tipped farther than normal and was putting extra strain on the ligaments which held it in place. He inserted a wire support gadget which helped hold the uterus in place and took the strain off the ligaments, and the ache cleared up. If she hadn't bothered to go see that one more doctor she could have easily started believing that the first few were right — that there was nothing wrong and that it was all *in her mind.*

I believe this is one of the general problems with backs. If a doctor tells you there is nothing wrong when you can't even bend over to tie your shoe, what are you supposed to think? I mean, doctors are supposed to *know,* right? They tell me its all in my mind, but it sure feels like its in my back! I'm not trying to fault the medical community here.

Doctors are human, for one thing, and they have to deal with a lot of complicated parts in a complex machine. And even a specialist dealing with back disorders can't necessarily *see* the pull or strain. Then again, maybe it *is* in your mind. So let's take a look at the difference between emotionally induced stress and psychosomatic disturbances. Or is there a difference?

One of the classic conditions which has been associated with emotional stress and tension is ulcers. An *ulcer personality,* or one who stands a high risk of developing ulcers, is the individual who faces a high degree of stress in the home or the workplace, who worries a lot and doesn't feel free to share that worry with others. One who, in general, holds emotions and concerns bottled up inside and has no satisfactory outlet for them. These emotional conditions generate bodily changes which can go on to create physical damage, in this case an ulcerated stomach. Other such emotionally induced conditions can include both a stiff neck and its resultant headache, and, I believe, a whole plethora of bodily ills, including backaches. These are accepted in many cases as stress oriented disorders, brought about in part or in whole by the mind and its emotions. And yet there is supposed to be a separate category of complaints labeled psychosomatic, which are supposed to be *real* only to the person doing the complaining. But there is a fine line here.

Psychosomatic disorders are supposed to be means of gaining attention, just like the child who intentionally does something wrong because a spanking is better than no attention at all, or of avoiding a situation that cannot be faced for whatever reason — *If my back is out I certainly can't be expected to attend that meeting I don't want to attend or solve that business problem that I can't seem to solve,* etc. Not necessarily on a conscious level, but the inner being providing an excuse for the self. And this is considered *not real,* compared to the *real* of the worry-induced ulcer or the stress-induced headache. Most clinicians will admit the pain seems real to the individual involved, but consider it unreal in the overall scheme of things. I believe the line is maybe a little too thin to try to differentiate between the two.

For example: If Businessman Bill has a problem he simply can't resolve satisfactorily, but has to answer for it to his boss on Friday morning, it appears very convenient and very *psychosomatic* for his back to go out Thursday night and be confined to bed for a few days. And many people will see it that way. I submit that perhaps Bill was experiencing so much frustration and tension during the previous days and weeks in trying to do the impossible, that the stress-induced tension in his back was tightening the muscles to a danger point. We have already seen how over-tight muscles can create strain in an area. Perhaps this strain got to the point in Bill's back where it pulled a ligament or tendon beyond its capability to extend. The resultant *attack* would smack heavily of being psychosomatic due to its timing, but would actually be a very real, stress-induced injury.

This same train may be put on the tracks of *just looking for affection* or *just needing some attention*. Such emotional needs can be very strong and, I believe, could certainly effect the body in a physical sense. Even though the primary source of therapy or treatment for these situations may need to be directed at the psychological or emotional needs of the individual, that is not to say that the fine line between psychosomatic and physical has not been crossed over, and that the immediate physical debility need not be addressed. It is my contention that in such cases the physical manifestations should be treated the same as any other injury (for that is what it is) and then look to the emotional cause to alleviate any future repeat performances.

8. OTHER — There are seemingly as many causes for back pain as there are functions of the body. These include, but are hardly limited to, kidney infections, stomach ulcers, a tipped uterus, prostate infections, menstruation, circulatory problems, tumors, abscesses, pneumonia, and the list

goes on. Even though the incidence of such *referred pains* are relatively uncommon in the overall scope of bad backs, it does point out the need for proper diagnosis to be sure that what is being treated is actually the cause, not just a symptom.

Chapter 3

LEANING

The most obvious physical manifestation associated with lower back pain is that of leaning. This is usually from the waist and can be just forward, but is usually a combination of a list to either port or starboard and a slight forward curling of the upper torso. Leaning is not simply an action to elicit sympathy from observers nor is it just an advance movement toward traveling in a particular direction. It is an involuntary posture brought about by the body attempting to minimize painful pressure upon a nerve root. As a temporary condition associated with some other primary painful condition of the spine, leaning is officially known as sciatic scoliosis, and consists of a spasm of muscles trying to protect the area that hurts. It may be brought about by a prolapsed disc or, as in my case, a pelvic hip joint contracture, among other causes. In any event, this form of scoliosis is temporary and will go away with correction of the underlying condition.

Regardless of what we call it, one of the most important lessons to learn about leaning is that if you lean when you walk, don't walk. When a back injury has advanced to the point of causing leaning, the best thing to do is stay in bed if at all possible, so as to not further aggravate the already existing muscle strain. Trying to be up and around while leaning not only worsens the existing problem but creates some very ungainly appearances. Its almost impossible, for example, to maintain a proper shirt tuck. The belt line will never be straight across the body and one shirt tail will inevitably crawl out in front creating a definitely derilict appearance. This very seldom ever impresses anyone and is best avoided whenever possible.

There are two methods I know of which may help temporarily correct the leaning syndrome. The first seems to be recommended by most health-care practitioners as it aids in straightening the spine and generally realigning the body structure. This is done simply by hanging vertically from a bar and allowing the body weight to gently pull the structure straight down. This can be pretty tough to do, depending on the severity of the trauma, but does aid in temporary realignment and relaxation of the back muscles which ordinarily have to support and balance the entire upper body weight. Obviously the bar height and security are very important to the success of this maneuver. You don't want the bar to be so high that you have to jump up to catch it, since you probably wouldn't be able to do that anyway. The bar also needs to be sturdy enough that you can be sure it won't slip and dump you unceremoniously, and painfully, on the floor.

There is a device on the market whereby you lean into a supported framework, have your ankles strapped securely onto the device, and are then revolved in a vertical, upside-down position to where your body weight is supported solely by your ankles. The same gravity realignment can then take place without the stress of having to support your weight with your hands. I have never had the opportunity to try one of these devices, so I am unable to recommend it personally, but the concept seems to make sense. I would suggest you discuss the possibility of such a device with your doctor.

The second method of temporary relief from leaning is not officially recommended as far as I know, but it is something I found, which helped me, so I will pass it along as a point of information.

When I leaned to the left I was usually able to somewhat comfortably lie on my right side, partially up on my right shoulder, because my back was then following the temporarily unnatural contour of my spine. I then rolled over carefully onto my back, relaxing the muscles as much as possible, and then slowly — and I mean slowly — on over to my left side. This provides a straighter alignment of the body, which runs contrary to the inclination of the back at the time, so it must be attempted gingerly and, oh, so cautiously.

If this position can be attained somewhat comfortably, the idea is then to raise the upper body slowly up onto the shoulder so that the body is bent or leaning in the opposite direction from which you started. This final maneuver can only be accomplished successfully with sufficient relaxation of the lower back muscles and should not be rushed by any stretch of the imagination. In fact, the entire operation of getting from one shoulder and direction to the other may take 10 or 15 minutes, perhaps longer.

If the trauma is severe enough, this maneuver may not be accomplished at all. Even if it is successful, you have basically only shifted the lean from one direction to another, but sometimes that is reward enough. The temporary relief of exchanging the strain from one set of muscles to another can be quite satisfying.

In general, the best rule concerning leaning is to heed it as a warning that something is wrong, receive treatment from your health-care practitioner, and stay off your feet to allow for proper healing.

Laughter creates an environment for healing.
Norman Cousins
Anatomy of an Illness

Chapter 4

A DAY IN THE COW PASTURE

Being a veteran back pain sufferer of many years, there is one phenomenon I am embarrassed to say wasn't brought to my attention until late in my *career*. During that phase of an episode when mobility was possible, although very uncomfortable, I had agreed to go out to the country with a friend to inspect a cow he was considering buying. After several days of being flat on my back the prospect of getting out of the house was very pleasant, but I had some apprehension as to how long I was going to last. The security of a readily available firm mattress had to be weighed against the frustration and isolation of a one-room existence. Finally fresh air won out and we were on our way.

Upon arriving at our destination, I was already experiencing the accumulation of every bump and pot hole encountered on our long ride through the back country roads. Before I could walk around the fields with any amount of effectiveness I had to stretch out as much as possible in the car to give my back a rest. After carefully maneuvering a six-foot-plus frame into a four-foot-minus space, I finally achieved a relatively comfortable position on my side —semi-prone, legs tucked, hips askance. I was just beginning to enjoy this temporary reprieve from pain when my friend came back to the car and said I looked like I was trying to flatulate out the window. Or words to that effect, anyway.

The realization suddenly hit me of the many strange and exotic positions back pain sufferers achieve in their constant quest of relief. How many meetings have we sat through continually squirming and fidgeting in our chairs trying to find a less uncomfortable position? Scooting forward and back on the seat, rocking from one cheek to the other, straightening, slumping, all in the elusive and innocent pursuit of comfort.

In retrospect I'm sure most of the unknowledgable observers thought we were either very blatant in our attempts to pass gas or were the not so proud possessors of some form of exotic tropical itch. I am now able to look back more knowledgably at the many raised eyebrows, behind-the-hand whisperings and, perhaps, intriguing rumors these actions must have elicited. But back to the cow pasture.

Once I had untangled from the car and regained my feet, I slowly followed my friend and the rancher into the field to find the subject cow. By this time I was almost glad I had chosen to take the trip. My back had been rested a little and it was a beautiful day. It was one of those days in New York's Adirondack Mountains that lifts the spirit and exhilerates the soul. The sky was a deep blue with only enough white fluffy clouds to give it character. A breeze was rustling through the stately pines and hardwoods stationed along the edge of the rolling pastures and the contented animals were peacefully grazing on the lush, green grass.

There was a feeling of serenity in the air, of a return to a more basic level of life and I was happy to be just where I was at that moment.

Happy, that is, until one of the *cows* not 20 feet from us began pawing the ground. Head lowered and menacing eyes staring straight at us, he began emitting a deep, rumbling noise from somewhere within his broad chest. I couldn't believe it! There we were, 2,000 miles from the nearest fence or building of any sort, confronted with the classic pose of a killer bull about to charge, obviously intent on wreaking havoc and destruction on any and all with which he came into contact.

A few moments before I had been glad to be alive. Now I had to look for a way to maintain that status.

Automatically my mind began to evaluate our position. Our trek out to this now desolate looking area had been a slow, arduous process as I had to watch my step not only for the usual reasons when crossing a pasture, but also to avoid the irregularities of the land contour. Trodding this uneven ground had increased the pain I was experiencing at a time when walking was difficult enough under ideal circumstances. And these were far from ideal circumstances.

Outrunning the creature was out of the question and the thought of trying to out-hobble a rampaging bull didn't seem very realistic. At one point the more imaginative portion of my mind conjured up images of leaping nimbly in the air over the bulky head, landing gracefully on the broad back and skillfully riding the beast until he stopped running out of frustration and fatigue. A sharp twinge in my back, however, immediately brought me back to reality and I dismissed this fantasy solution to my dilemma.

When faced with seemingly imminent danger a person usually has two available responses: engage the enemy or retreat. Since the latter appeared impractical and the former impossible, I opted for a third choice. I tried to ignore the problem and hoped like hell it would go away. Which, in a way, is exactly what happened.

No, the bull didn't leave. In fact, he stayed right where he was and continued to paw the ground and bellow all the time we were there. Our host, in the meantime, was paying little attention to this dramatic sideshow. At one point he said in an offhand manner, "Don't worry about the bull, he probably won't do anything." That's supposed to be reassuring? Probably? It *probably* won't rain the day of our picnic; the T.V. *probably* won't break down during the final two minutes of the Super Bowl; our nation's currency will *probably* last and I will *probably* live at least another 40 years. Then I realized that what he meant was *when* the bull attacked *they* could *probably* make it to safety because

I would be left behind as a hobbling human sacrifice to the lord of the field. A poor, pathetic creature destined to be stomped and smashed into a messy little spot resembling nothing more than one of the cow flops with which the pasture was so liberally decorated.

This little experience, however, did have a happy, if not dramatic, ending. When finally I could take the pressure no longer and my back was tightening like a clenched fist, I forcibly joined the conversation and immediately turned and started walking Grandpa McCoy style back to the barn. Fortunately my companions fell for it and accompanied me slowly back across the field, chatting amicably, as if it were simply time to go back to the house to tie down the deal. They didn't understand that I was *running for my life.*

Even though I was verbally part of the conversation, I have no idea what was discussed. I was much too busy keeping one eye on the uneven ground in front of me and the other on the bull behind. To this day I'm sure neither my friend nor our host realize how close we came to death on that warm, sunny afternoon in the cow pasture.

Chapter 5

EXERCISE

Good physical health and body conditioning is one of the major elements in avoiding debilitating back problems. That is not to say that the finely tuned athlete won't ever suffer from a back strain or injury, because they will. Anyone who follows the NFL is well aware of John Riggens' past practice of weekly hospital stays in traction to be able to play on the weekend. But assuming you are not a running back for the Redskins, a good general conditioning exercise program can help decrease — and maybe eliminate — the incidence of your back troubles.

The reason for this is quite simple: our muscles are designed to be used and will function better if they are kept in running order. Speaking of running, perhaps a word of caution would be appropriate here. Physical fitness is becoming quite a fad today. In every park in the country you can see people running back and forth or 'round and 'round, as the case may be. Aerobics programs are popping up everywhere and many people are dashing off to health clubs to play with the machines. I'm not saying there's anything wrong with this at all, just keep in mind we are talking physical fitness, not fanaticism. I feel the popular *no pain, no gain* is being grossly overused and overrated. Just because it may be good to run a mile or two doesn't mean its better to run a hundred. Forty reps on a machine aren't necessarily twice as good as twenty. We are trying to *use* our muscles, not *abuse* them.

I realize physical fitness can be quite a social endeavor. Working out in the right club or running in the correct jogging apparel can be beneficial...to our economy. Personally I get a real kick out of seeing someone drive to the club to work out or take a cab to the park so they can run. We seem to spend so much money avoiding work — having the lawn mowed, the walk shoveled and the leaves raked — that we have to spend more to get our *exercise*. Sometimes doing what comes naturally is not only less expensive, but much more rewarding.

In any event, whatever your preference in fashion and lifestyle, keep in mind the frequency of your activities. Just as with whole bran fibre, regularity is the key. An occasional binge of physical activity is asking for trouble to an otherwise sedentary body. The company's annual softball game is almost guaranteed to produce an injury to the individual who rides a desk the other 364 days of the year. Whatever you do to get your exercise, try to do it two or three times a week. Your muscles will appreciate it and so, ultimately, will you.

Now that I have preached my own philosophy on exercise in general, perhaps I should become more specific as to the point of this chapter — exercises for the individual with a bad back.

Certain mild exercises can be performed by persons suffering from back pain to help align the body and strengthen muscles which assist in body stability. These maneuvers are not meant to build the body beautiful or to give you the edge over the sand-kicking beach bully. They will, however, help keep you on your feet or get you back on your feet sooner. And after all, that's what this book is all about.

Needless to say, you won't have to travel to the local gym to perform these exercises, nor is there any special equipment necessary. I will outline several such exercises which may be performed in bed.

MODIFIED SIT-UPS: The purpose in sit-ups generally is to strengthen the stomach muscles. For those with bad backs, a firm set of stomach muscles is advantageous

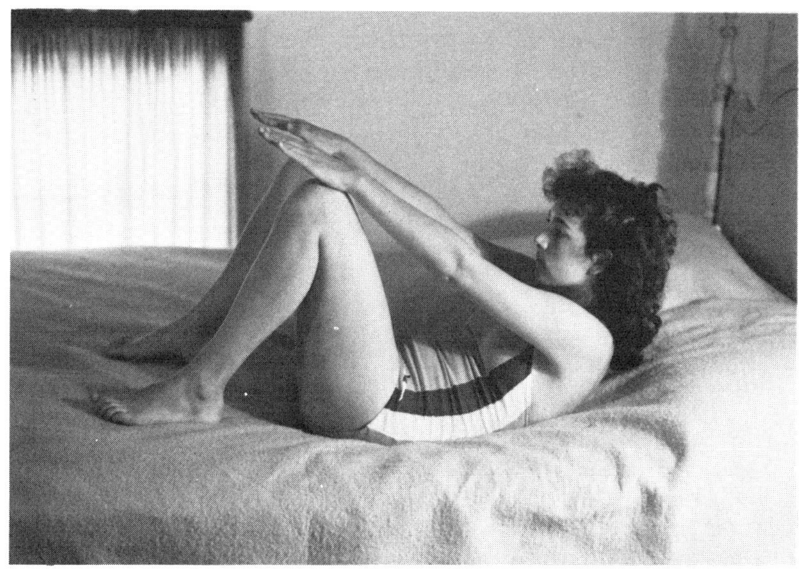

MODIFIED SIT-UPS. This avoids the extra pull in the lower back found with regular sit-ups, but still exercises the stomach muscles. You won't impress any friends by trying to show-off with these modified sit-ups, but you can certainly build a good fire in your belly if you do them correctly.

for more than being able to catch a medicine ball without keeling over. They are an integral part of the overall body alignment. If you are carrying some extra pounds in a saggy belly, that weight is carried out in front of the body which requires back muscles to compensate to hold the body erect. As has already been covered, any time the back muscles have to compensate for the body being out of balance, there may be hell to pay later.

Lying flat on your back, knees elevated, extend your arms forward and slowly curl the upper part of your body forward until your wrists come close to touching your knees. Curl back down to a prone position and repeat the procedure until you feel a pull in your stomach muscles. As with any exercise, repetition is better than overexertion. You can always come back and do some more of these later, so don't try to set your belly on fire the first time out. Important: in lifting the upper body, be sure to roll your body forward, starting with your head and shoulders. Do not try to lift straight up from the waist as is done with regular sit-ups. Raise only the upper body, and then only enough to make the contact of wrist to knee.

Note: According to Dr. Rowland Hazard of the New England Back Center, new findings indicate that firm stomach muscles may not play as major a role in helping back pains as was once thought. Since a flat stomach feels better than a saggy one, however, I still recommend this exercise.

KNEE LIFTS: All of these exercises are performed while lying on your back, so I shall dispense with repeating that part of the instructions.

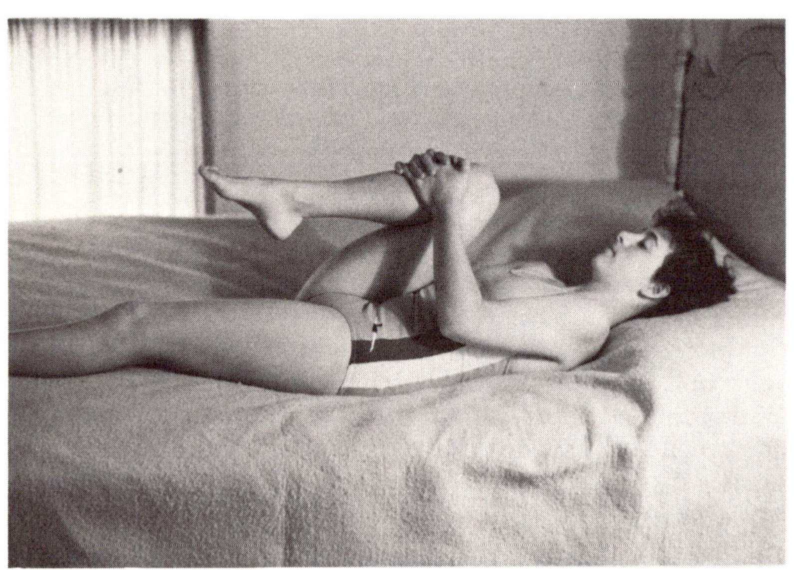

KNEE LIFTS. Rotate your hips when changing legs on this one and you will feel the relaxation taking place in your lower back. A great loosener.

Knee lifts are designed to develop lower back flexibility and assist in hip alignment.

Keeping one leg extended, raise the other knee to a point where you may reach it with both hands. Lock your fingers around the knee and gently pull the leg toward your upper body. I say pull gently and that's exactly what I mean. You want to develop a slight muscle loosening in your lower back, not rip the leg from its socket. Lower that leg to the extended position and repeat the performance with the other leg. Repeat these sets, pulling only a little harder with each set. There is no fixed number of repetitions for this exercise and it is not designed to tire any particular muscle, so there will be no obvious stopping point from exertion. Repeat until you feel a little relaxation in the hips and lower back, then rest a while.

When performing the knee lifts, try to develop a slight hip rotation when changing legs. The hip on the side of the leg being lifted should be slightly rotated down toward the feet. I have found this hip shift is best accomplished with both legs extended, slowly, while changing from one knee to the other.

LEG CROSS: This exercise is also designed to develop extra mobility in the lower back and help align the hips. You remember alignment? I may have mentioned it before and I'm sure I will again, because its one of the keys to this whole operation.

Picture your body and its skeletal structure as one of the sets of scales used in the portrayal of blind justice. You know the kind, a vertical bar with a crossbar containing a cup or plate at either end for holding the weights and item to be weighed. Now picture your spine as the vertical bar with the part of the crossbar being played by your pelvis. The cups or plates at either end of the crossbar are, of course, your hip sockets.

Just as the crossbar in the scales goes down on one side as the weight is increased, so does your pelvis rotate as your upper body weight is shifted. The only problem is that

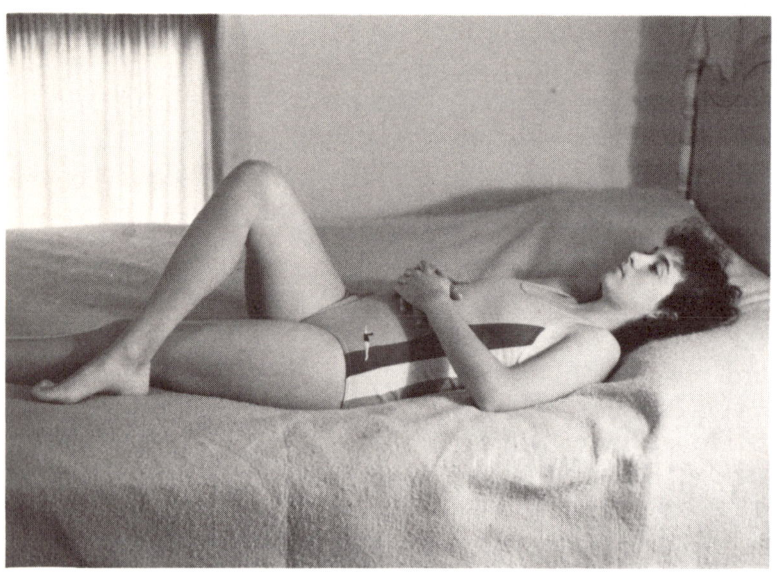

LEG CROSS. *After sliding one foot up to the other knee (above), allow the raised leg to lower toward the bed of its own weight (below). Just relax and let it go, do not force the knee down.*

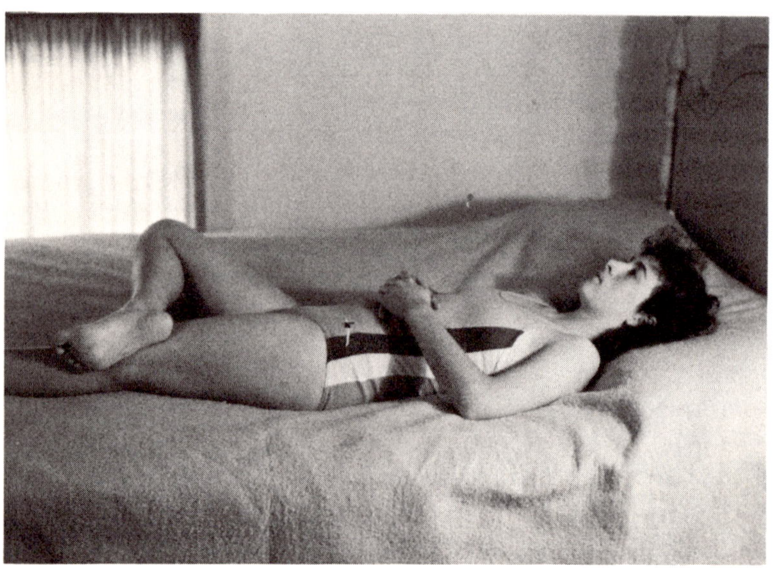

your entire upper body weight is being supported and balanced by the pelvis which, in turn, is connected to your spine by a series of ligaments and muscles. When everything is in balance or rotating up and down freely, there is little problem. But when the spine or vertical bar is out of alignment or the pelvis or crossbar is tilted too far to one side for too long, the rest of the structure has to take over to reestablish balance. These muscles and ligaments can then be overworked and stretched and may become inflamed and swollen. As you know, any muscle which is overworked tends to cramp up. Voila! Back spasms.

Now, back to our leg cross exercise. With legs extended, cross one ankle over the other. Slowly slide the topside foot up to where the ankle is above the knee of the lower leg. Now lower the raised knee sideways, down toward the mattress. Again, you will feel a slight pull in your lower back, and perhaps in your hips as well. Do not force your leg down. This could defeat the benefit of the exercise. Simply allow the weight of your knee to do the pulling while you keep your entire body relaxed. When it feels like you have achieved a slight stretch in your back, raise your knee to about 45 degrees and slide your foot back to the extended position, using the lower leg for support. Repeat the process with your other leg.

These last two exercises — the Knee Lift and Leg Cross — are what I have found to work best for me at those times when my back feels cranky. Old timers might call it *all stoved up,* but it really makes no difference, a few repetitions of these and my back feels looser and much better.

KNEE CROSS: Unlike the leg cross, this one starts with knees elevated. Cross your right leg over the left as if you were crossing your legs in a chair. Using the weight of your right leg, gently lower the left leg down to the right. The ultimate goal is to touch the bed or floor with the left knee while keeping your upper back flat. If there is too much tightness, don't fight it, just stretch it a little and return to the starting position. Reverse the process and use your left

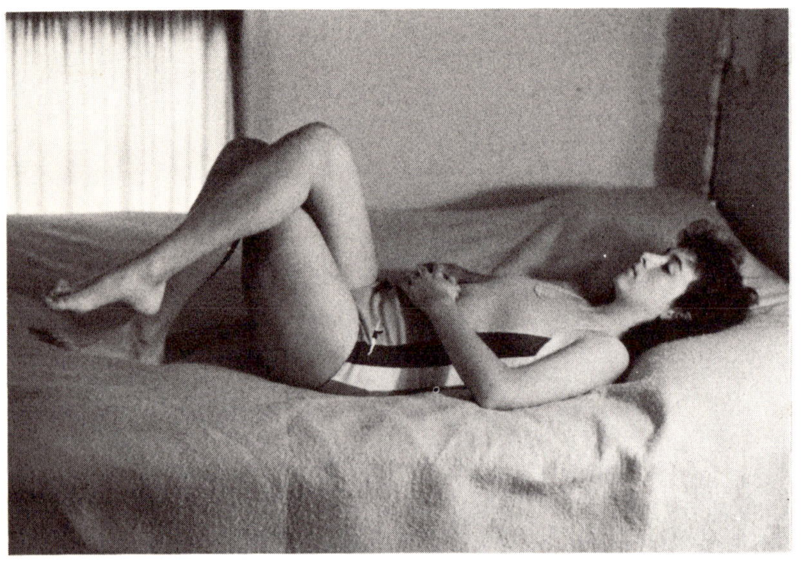

KNEE CROSS. The same principle applies here as with the LEG CROSS. Another great relaxer and loosener.

leg to pull your right leg down to the side. Careful stretching will allow you to go a little further with each repetition, so don't push it. Do this a few times to each side and then relax a while. As with any of these exercises, don't try to go too far too fast.

PELVIC TILT: This is a fairly new one to me and it sounded terrible when I first heard about it, but it does seem to help. All you have to do is lie on your back with knees elevated and tighten your buttocks for a few seconds. What this will do is raise your pelvis slightly and flatten your spine down to the surface on which you are lying. Again, it helps stretch the muscles in your lower back to reduce the tightness. Don't intentionally try to flatten your spine, just squeeze your buttocks together as hard as you can for a few seconds and let the pelvis tilt by itself, then relax. Do a few repetitions and treat yourself to any kind of fantasy you wish.

Keep in mind these exercises are not meant to develop bulging biceps or build a "V" shaped torso. They are stretching and limbering maneuvers, the same as any athlete performs before going into more strenuous activities. And if you happen to be a jock and feel ridiculous doing such *sissy* exercises, remember that while you may ordinarily be able to run a four-minute mile or lift a truck, right now you probably can't lift your own body off the bed or run across the room. So why not give them a try? They might just help get you back on your feet so you can go reconquer the world.

WHY FIX THE ROOF NOW? IT'S NOT RAINING.

The exercises outlined in this chapter are designed for use during episodes of back pain. They are very helpful

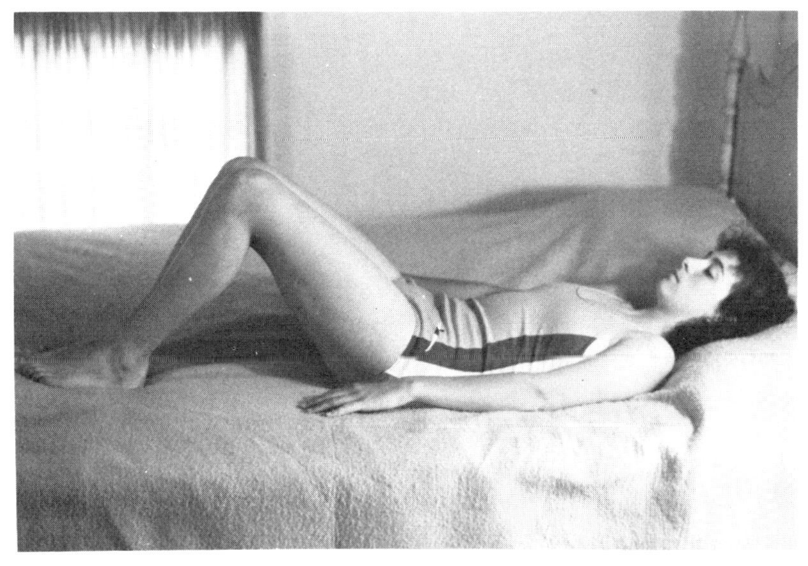

PELVIC TILT. Simply tighten the buttocks and allow the pelvis to tilt up. I know it doesn't look as if much is going on here, but it does feel good when done correctly.

during such times of decreased mobility, but should not be thought of as the final solution to back problems. They are only the patch to the roof when it is raining. The best time to combat back troubles is when it is *not* raining. This means developing and maintaining positive emotional and physical living patterns while you are healthy, not waiting for something to go wrong and then trying to catch up. Learn to more effectively control the stress situations in your life, relax when you may, and practice a continuing program of regular physical exercise.

There are several good exercise programs on the market which have been designed for individuals with back problems. Several of them are listed in the bibliography of this book and I'm sure your local bookstore would be glad to get them for you if they are not in stock. Check with your doctor to see what would be best for your age group and physical condition.

There is a general exercise program on the market which was designed specifically for senior citizens. It was produced by Stacy Keach, Sr. after having undergone open heart surgery. When I asked him about it he said it was developed by a team of leading cardiologists and exercise physiologists and is designed to strengthen the heart, increase energy, relax tension and lose or redistribute weight. Sounds a lot like what we have just been discussing, doesn't it? This program is called *Approved Exercises for Senior Citizens* and is available from Stacy Keach Productions, 5216 Laurel Danyon Boulevard, North Hollywood, California, 91607. Or you can give him a call at 213-877-0472.

Whatever you do, don't wait until it rains to think about that hole in the roof. Just as it is much more enjoyable to work outside on a warm, sunny afternoon, it is much easier to maintain good health than to have to try to regain it later.

Chapter 6
SEX, MEDICATION &
THE SNEEZE

SEX

Even though the sex drive may be reduced somewhat during a severe bout of back pain, that doesn't mean it won't make its presence known from time to time. Since cold showers and long walks are probably not advisable under the circumstances, there may be some good news for you here. In many cases the main problem of having sex while experiencing back pain is the fear of the pain itself. While severe back problems can sometimes cause or contribute to impotency in men and frigidity in women because of the threat of expected pain, it has been found medically (and personally) that if done right, the gentle pelvic thrusts of intercourse can in fact be good therapy for a poor back. Besides for providing physical and emotional pleasure and satisfaction, it can reduce the stress and tension, which may actually be contributing to the pain you are experiencing.

We have found already that many elements interact within the human body and psyche to form what appears to be a single manifestation, in this case, back pain. We have seen (or will see) how relaxation of mind and body can reduce the level of pain experienced and contribute to the healing process. In the case of sex we are dealing with a whole range of physical and emotional needs — touch, intimacy, reassurance, satisfaction and movement. If nothing else we have a form of exercise with real motivation.

One element which may need mentioning here is that of trust and understanding between the partners. If your partner understands the fear aspect involved for you and you can trust him/her to not become too rambunctious, you are then free to proceed at your own pace with expectation rather than apprehension. If you are not sure your partner fully appreciates your position, talk to them. Talking is easy and doesn't cost a dime. Lord knows I do enough of it.

Now that we have established that sex with a bad back is probably okay, and maybe even desirable, what positions may best be assumed?

This is a question you will have to answer for yourself. You may find you are still capable of the exotic maneuverings of the most athletic and adventurous. And maybe not. If not, take heart, there is still hope.

Probably the easiest is the *spoon* position where both partners are on their sides facing the same direction with knees bent, and the man is cupped into the woman's back. This not only provides good access but has the advantage of equal weight distribution along the entire body. Second choice would be on the sides, facing. This has the same advantage of weight distribution but the disadvantage of needing legs over and under other legs, thereby creating a realignment of the spine which may be uncomfortable. Male superior, female superior, female astride and mounted position all require some individual support and have the possibility of an unexpected weight shift which may be most distressing if encountered suddenly.

The sexual activity you and your partner may enjoy during back pain is pretty much an individual matter. You will soon discover by experimentation what works best for you. Reason would say to take things slowly and don't try to be too acrobatic, but if you still have your heart set on the *hanging basket* or *whirling dirvish,* good luck and may God bless you.

MEDICATION

Even if I were a physician, which I am not, I trust I would have the presence of mind to not prescribe medication through such a general medium as a book. Medication should be taken only after being advised by a competent medical practitioner for a specific, known condition. Even over-the-counter drugs and pain relievers may do more harm than good when taken on a self-prescribed basis.

The problem here is that pain is an indication that something is wrong somewhere in the body. It may be involved in the area in which the pain is felt and it may not. Doctors call this *referred pain* when, for whatever reason, a malady in the body will manifest its sensation elsewhere. A classic example of this is sciatica, where pain radiates down a leg, but the disturbance is actually up in the hip area. Taking self-prescribed medication for an undiagnosed condition can temporarily mask the symptoms while leaving the original disruption to possibly worsen. Simply masking a pain is usually desired, but not always beneficial.

I remember as a youngster asking my parents why we have to feel pain. The answer I received at the time is the same one I gave my children 25 years later, "It helps you know when something is wrong in your body." All I knew at the time, however, was that pain hurt and I didn't like it one bit. I didn't see why we couldn't have little warning lights or buzzers that would go off telling us it was time for something to be repaired somewhere. I didn't realize, of course, that if we did have just warning lights, how easy it would be to put off the repairs to a more convenient time. We are too inclined to do the term paper in the wee hours of the final day or replace the fan belt after it breaks. Apparently we need the incentive of wanting to stop the pain to get us to do something about the problem. Its really not a bad system, actually, when you realize it could save your life.

So pay attention to those warning lights that demand your immediate attention. Remember they aren't just annoyances, they are trying to tell you something which may be important. Find out what they are saying and take care of it. Don't just mask the message and pretend its not there.

THE SNEEZE

Short of being trampled by the bull in Chapter Five or tossed around the room by a professional wrestler, probably the single most fearful occurrence facing someone whose back is out is a sneeze. You can picture it, right? You're lying in bed minding your own business when suddenly your nose starts to itch. *Oh God, why me? I try to lead a good life. I don't mug old ladies, I take vitamin "C" everyday and I've never robbed a single bank in my entire life. Why do I have to sneeze at this particular time? Next week would do just fine!*

But the itch grows. You rub your nose until you think it might break, and the itch grows. You try to smother yourself with a pillow thinking that even if you can't stop the sneeze you might just be able to die before it hits. Since there is seldom enough time to suffocate before the sneeze, however, the best you can do is try to reduce the velocity of the explosion and brace yourself for the worst.

In my experience, this is best accomplished by bending your knees and making sure that as much of your weight as possible is supported. If you are standing, flex your knees, bend over and support your torso by placing hands on knees. If you are in bed, even better. Raise your knees to take any additional strain off the lower back. The best I have found, however, is to roll onto your side and assume a fetal position. This offers the same advantage as the spoon position during sex of providing maximum weight support to reduce as much of the impact as possible. A sneeze or severe cough puts a tremendous amount of sudden stress on the muscles of the back which is just what they don't need right at this time.

If you happen to be fortunate enough to sneeze like my sister-in-law who produces nothing more than a series of little *choos*, then perhaps you have a chance of survival. In the case of the rafter-rockers, like me, the involuntary muscle contractions necessary to generate a resounding aaaaCHOO! will create a veritable explosion of white pain which starts from the existing spasm and radiates out through the very soul. Not a pleasant situation, at best.

Unfortunately I know of no guaranteed remedies for this problem. You might try outlawing pepper from your house or having the air vaccuumed continuously to rid it of dust. But ultimately, if it happens, it happens, and the best you can do is minimize the impact and hope it doesn't happen again until you are well.

Of course this does create possibilities for the more evil-minded of individuals. For example: John was recuperating from a hernia repair when Richard brought him a joke book to read. The following year when Richard was healing from an adult circumcision, John brought in a Playboy magazine. Let's see...a vial of sneezing powder for a friend laid up with a bad back...no! No hatred could run that deep.

An individual develops pain in his back as a defense mechanism in a situation in which he finds he can no longer cope with emotional difficulties...

Leon Root, MD
Hospital of Special Surgery
New York City
Author of *Oh, My Aching Back*

Chapter 7

WHAT ABOUT CHIROPRACTIC?

In the field of treatment and healing there are several disciplines which apply to back problems. These are generally broken down into three health-care providers: allopathic (medical), chiropractic and osteopathic. Since back injuries may apply to any of the three groups, depending upon the injury, I will not recommend one above the others. I will, in fact, suggest that anyone suffering from frequent and severe back pains consult with each of the groups for diagnosis and recommended treatment. Just as the health community in general is suggesting second opinions, I strongly suggest a second and even third opinion be obtained. This is especially true before commencement of a possibly major treatment program. You wouldn't buy the first car offered for sale or accept the first investment program presented, would you? Well, I believe you also should not accept the first diagnosis as fact or *buy* the treatment program that sounds easiest or is cheapest. This is your health we are discussing here and it behooves you to get additional information before deciding on treatment.

I said I would not recommend any of the three fields of health care above the others, and now I am going to spend a little space expounding on the practice of chiropractic. The reason for this is simple — it is what I found works for me, for my particular situation. Perhaps a spot of background is appropriate here.

As I have mentioned, I suffered from frequent episodes of debilitating back pain for over 20 years. During that time I saw five or six medical doctors, one chiropractor and an osteopath. The diagnoses I received ranged from the mundane to the frightful and recommended treatments ran from aspirin to surgery. Short of having surgery, none of the treatments helped very much. It got to the point where I was expecting to simply live with the periodic bouts for the rest of my life.

Then in the fifth week of a major experience, my wife talked me into calling a second chiropractor who had been highly endorsed by friends. I wasn't especially enthusiastic as I felt the first chiropractor I had seen some 18 years before had done little to help. But I was desperate for some relief, any relief, from the constant pain which had kept me bedridden for over a month and which was beginning to effect my outlook on life. If you have been through one of these experiences, you know what I'm talking about. At first you're afraid you're going to die. As time grinds on you are afraid you won't. Walking is excruciating, if possible at all. The high point of a day is to find a position which doesn't hurt quite as much as the rest, and the immediate objective is to be able to finally nod off for a few hours of fitfull sleep. All things considered, not an enjoyable situation. I was ready to try anything.

Since I was unable to leave the house, Charles Spaulding, Doctor of Chiropractic, came over that afternoon. That was my first surprise. The second surprise was when he diagnosed my problem as hips out of alignment. Okay, I hadn't heard *that* one before, but who was I to argue? He also said that due to the extent of the trauma it would take a few sessions to get everything back in order. That one I *was* expecting. The third and most pleasant surprise, however, came just two days and as many treatments later when I found myself back on my feet and feeling great. That was four years ago at the time of this writing. Since then I have had a few threatening episodes which Dr. Spaulding has nipped in the bud.

Am I saying by this example that chiropractic is a miracle cure and osteopaths and medical doctors are frauds? No, far from it. All doctors are highly skilled individuals trained to cope with a myriad of injuries, illnesses and just plain complaints. The reason for the emergence of specialists is that no one individual can be expected to know everything about all ailments of the human body. There are certainly instances with back pain which will require the attention of an osteopath or surgeon. That's the reason for suggesting a second opinion. There are also a great many situations, in my opinion, where the skills of a good chiropractor may offer satisfying results.

Chiropractic, by definition, is "a system of therapeutics based upon the theory that disease is caused by interference with nerve function, the method being to restore normal condition by adjusting body structures, esp. the spinal column." As discussed in the chapter on the back, this spinal column consists of 24 vertebrae separated by 23 discs. The discs act as shock absorbers and allow movement of the spine, but may sometimes slip or become compressed by injury. Down through this stack of vertebrae and discs travel 31 pairs of spinal nerves which serve every living tissue of the body. The problem with some back conditions is that because of the complicated network of nerves traveling through the spinal column, the pain may manifest itself some distance from the actual injury.

A leaky roof is sometimes difficult to pin down as to the exact location of the leak because the entering water will often travel an extensive course of rafters and joists before making its appearance in the ceiling. Until the cause of the leak is discovered, the best we can do is place a pan or two around to catch the drips. In the case of back pains, ointments and heat treatments are often nothing more than catching the drips. If a spinal nerve root is pressured or irritated by a displacement or derangement of one or more of the vertebrae, addressing the pain which may be manifest elsewhere is only treating the symptom, not the cause. Chiropractors, by adjusting the affected area, seek to alle-

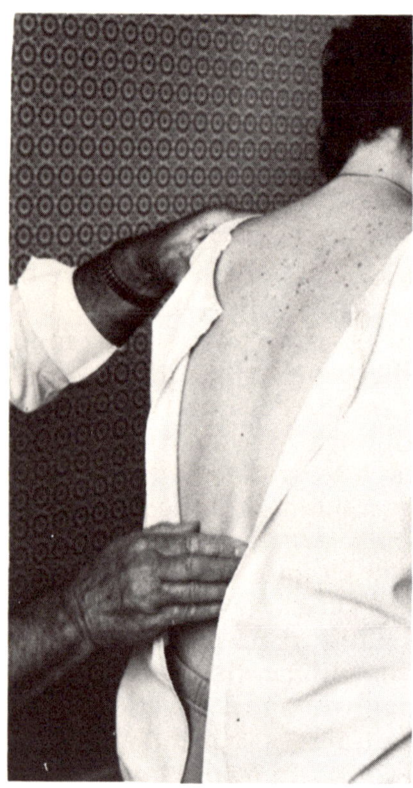

A spinal exam by a doctor of chiropractic. It is this examination and concentration on the spine which sets chiropractors apart from other health practitioners.

viate the *cause* of the spinal nerve irritation rather than simply treat the symptom. And once the cause has been remedied, we can put our drip pans — and heating pads — away.

Contrary to some popular beliefs, chiropractors are not *bone crackers*. Whereas there may in fact be some popping sounds heard during a manipulation treatment, these are nothing more than the cracking of a knuckle which often brings relief and restores flexibility to the joint. It may sound terrible, but it doesn't hurt.

My infrequent visits to Dr. Spaulding always start with a spinal exam while seated. This consists of his feeling the placement of the vertebrae along the spine. He then

What About Chiropractic?

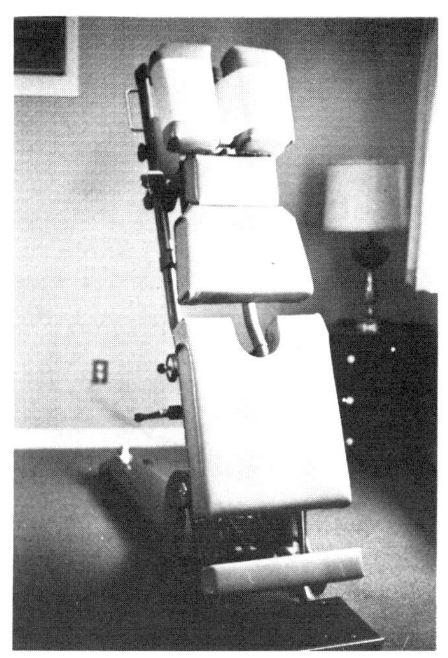

A chiropractic treatment table in the raised position. This enables a patient to simply lean into the table and be lowered gently to the working position (below), rather than having to climb onto a fixed table height which can be very difficult to do with a painful back. Note the various openings and adjustments available to help assure comfort. All in all, a very interesting piece of machinery.

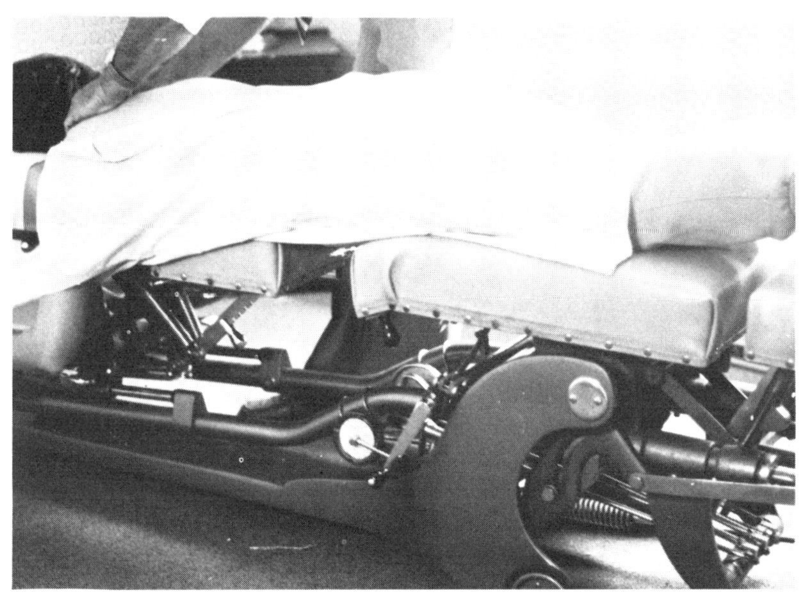

checks the balance of my hips while standing, and we proceed to the treatment table. As you see in the illustrations, the table is not something which must be climbed onto. That could be very difficult at times. It is an adjustable device which can be made to fit different body sizes and which is raised to a near vertical position so that you need merely to lean into it. It is then lowered to the horizontal position with the aid of counter-balancing springs or weights.

The treatment includes a series of physical manipulations to correct the position of the vertebrae, realign the hips, straighten the spine or whatever may be appropriate for the individual. There is very little, if any, pain, and it

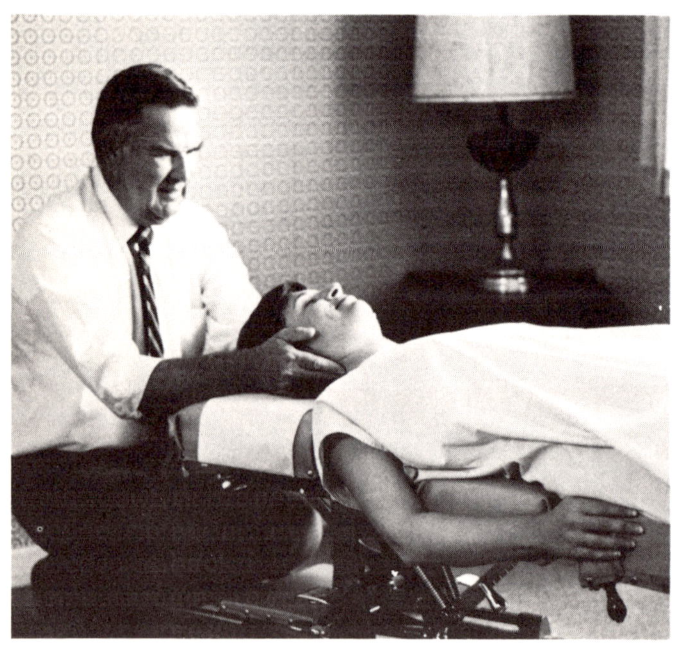

Dr. Charles Spaulding at work. He is the man responsible for getting me back on my feet and keeping me there. Thanks, Charlie.

can be quite relaxing. I will not describe any of the manipulations in detail as they are designed to be performed by trained professionals for specific purposes. What may be helpful to one situation may be damaging to another and none should be performed on an amateur basis any more than medications should be self-prescribed. If you see a chiropractor he or she will decide what is best for you.

Initial chiropractic visits may sometimes require x-rays to rule out the existence of bone fractures, tumors, etc. And if a more serious situation is discovered, you will probably be referred on to a specialist for treatment. In most cases, however, a good chiropractor will have you up and around before long, and feeling better than ever.

Some opponents of manipulation claim that the *laying on of hands* combined with the attention to patient education and ongoing longitudinal care so often displayed by chiropractors, is as important as the manipulation maneuvers themselves. And this may in fact be the case. If it is, perhaps the practitioners of manipulation have rediscovered a basic tenent of medicine which some physicians today seem to have forgotten — that the healing process is greatly assisted by a little care and attention on the part of the practitioner. We are, after all, human beings with fears and apprehensions, not simply machines taken to a shop for repair.

A couple of statistics from the back patient survey show an interesting correlation between the attitude of the practitioner and the results as perceived by the patient. Of those visiting a chiropractor, 69% of the individuals felt the practitioner indicated a caring attitude and 71% of those felt the result of that treatment were satisfactory or better. For medical visits, 56% felt the attitude was caring, which produced only 48% of satisfactory or better results. While this survey is far from scientific, and it would be wonderful to see 100% results across the board, it is interesting to see a relationship between the practitioner's attitude and the results as perceived by the patient.

Along this line, I would like to close this chapter with

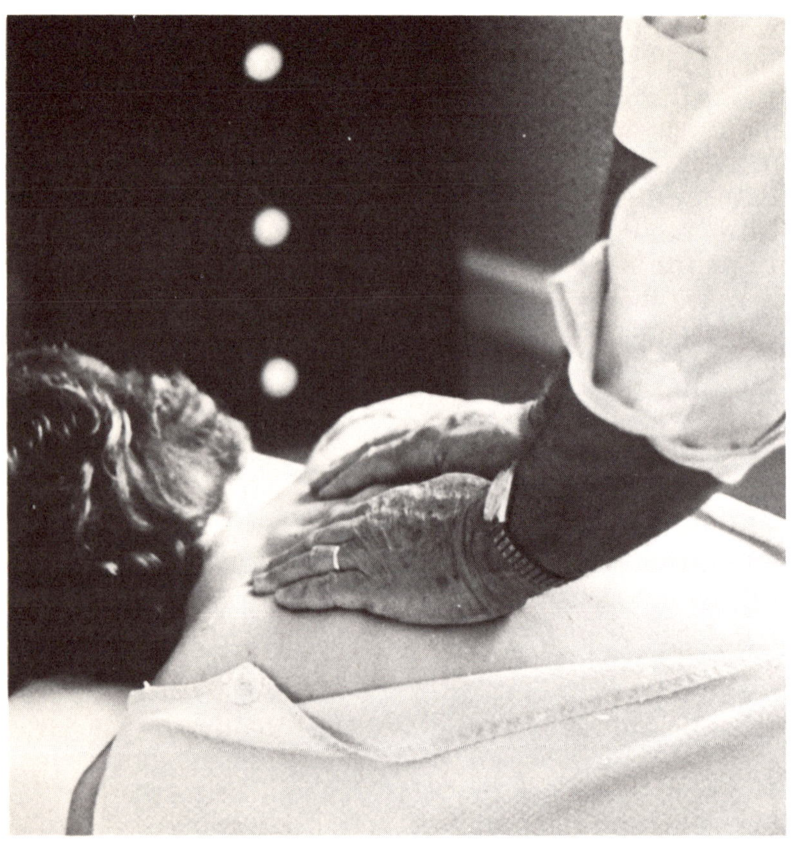

Simple massage or laying on of hands? Many opponents of chiropractic feel these are the main benefits of manipulation treatment. Although there is a lot to be said about the therapeutic value of the interaction between practitioner and patient, there is much more to it than that. A chiropractic adjustment by Dr. Spaulding puts things back where they belong and allows me to go on with my life, free of pain.

a personal message to any of the other 30-40% of health-care practitioners who may be reading this. I understand that oftentimes your patient load may be overwhelming and I appreciate the fact that you are doing your best with a little-understood malady, but please keep in mind that while for you our visit is only one more in an otherwise full day, for us it is our *only* visit of the day, and is very important. We are all aware of the occasional value of a placebo. I suggest that sometimes just a little extra care and attention on your part will go a long way to assist our recovery.

Chapter 8

THE SOCK

The self-application of clothing for one suffering from lower back pain is a difficulty which needs to be experienced to be appreciated. Most of it may be accomplished with a little patience, a lot of tooth gritting and a few hints garnered from more years of experience than I like to remember. Most of it, that is, except *the sock*. Anyone who has never tried putting on socks when they were incapable of even coming close to touching either foot will probably want to skip this chapter as everything related here will be outside their scope of experience. For those of you still reading, lets take things in order.

Upper body clothing presents no particular problem. Anyone experiencing back pain, and who still has the need and motivation to get dressed, can accomplish the application of shirts, jackets, coats and, I suppose, bras with no more than a little patient maneuvering. The items may not hang properly when placed, but will at least have the wearer more or less ready to face the public from the waist up.

Pants present a little more of a challenge, but may be installed either from a horizontal or vertical position. If horizontal, simply position the garment at the foot of the bed (or floor) with the leg holes pointing at your feet. The placing of the garment at the extreme end of your body will take some time, but where there is determination there is a method. Once the leg holes are positioned, a little skillful maneuvering of the toes, one leg at a time, will gain access of the garment. From that point it is only a matter of time and slow squiggling downward until the top of the pants can be reached by hand. By slowly rolling from one cheek to the other, the pants may then be inched upward to the waistline and be considered close enough for fastening.

In the case of a vertical application of pants, being a *leaner* has a distinct advantage. Holding the garment by one side of the waistband, stretch your leaning arm downward so that the hanging leg opening approaches the point of access, i.e. that point at which the toes of one foot may be carefully wriggled into the opening. The second foot is a little more complicated but requires only a little careful maneuvering of one foot in concert with the other, already placed foot, until both feet are firmly ensconced in the appropriate leg holes. (This operation usually requires the assistance of a headboard or dresser to support the very tenously balanced position.) The remainder of the task simply entails the careful inching upwards of the pants until they reach their appointed position.

Don't be overly concerned with trying to attain a tailored-appearance shirt tuck. Crooked belt lines and flapping shirt tails during such times are becoming more socially acceptable than a few years ago. Remember, you have already avoided being arrested for indecent exposure and are fortunate enough to be on your feet, so its all frosting on the cake from here.

Shoes take a close second to hats in ease of installation. The reason for this is that anyone who has experienced even one bout of low back pain should know enough to keep a pair of loafers or slip-ons around the house. It goes without saying that the footwear should be large enough to slip on easily unless you keep a three-foot shoe horn around the house.

This inevitably brings us back to our archenemy, *the sock*. On this item I have a special request to make of those of you outside our circle of experience. The next time you witness a poor mortal listing to starboard or port and hobbling slowly across a street or a living room wearing loafers over otherwise bare feet, have a little compassion, for you will soon learn why they are thusly attired.

Picture yourself sitting obliquely on your bed with a sock in each hand meant to go on feet you cannot so much as touch. Due to the interrelated (and painful) musculature of your back, you cannot bend your torso down or your legs up enough to make the contact of hand to foot. *The sock* is much too small and too limp to place on the floor and wriggle into as may be done with pants. Again, if you are a *leaner,* you may be able to install the little critter on one foot or the other, and your problem is halfway resolved. Or is it? If you are rich enough to be considered eccentric, you will probably get away with it. But for the rest of us, to appear in public with one socked foot and one naked foot is hardly better than two bare feet, all things considered.

So, what do you do? I'm sorry to report that I have no easy answers. If you are married your spouse will probably assist in this matter. If you are wealthy you could hire someone to come in each morning and put your socks on for you. However, if you are poor and single or have an unwilling spouse, either stay in the house or go *Bohemian.*

Chapter 9

BACK SUPPORTS

The majority of individuals in today's society spend all of their daily allotment of 24 hours in one of three positions — standing, sitting and lying. We may occasionally encounter the squatting position so prevelant in Third World countries (where the incidence of back problems is said to remain low, by the way) and the kneeling position so favored by Victorian romance writers, but these are by so far the exception they will not be considered further here.

Ours is a sedentary society. The root meaning of sedentary is *to sit*. And sit, we do. We have made such great strides in technology over the last century that most of us are no longer subject to the *backbreaking* work which was so common to our forebears. We are now able to sit at work, sit at meals, sit in the car and sit at home. We sit in stadiums and bleachers watching our favorite team exert and compete. We can even sit at typewriters telling others how much we sit. We have reduced the need for physical activity to the point where most of us spend more time sitting than in both of the other two positions combined. And we are damaging our backs in the process.

Pressure on the spinal discs is increased when seated. This is because the spine is no longer being supported by the muscles of our back, but is instead subject to the contour of the chair or seat against which it is leaning. And the fact is that most chairs and seats today are simply not designed to afford proper support. While this issue is currently being addressed by the seating industry, we cannot shunt all the blame off to the manufacturers. We are encouraging the continuation of poor design by paying more attention (and money) to the choice of fabric or color than to the support design of the unit being offered. The result of this selection process is that the chairs and seats in which we spend so much of our time are doing us more harm than good.

One remedy for this is to do less sitting and develop a more physically active lifestyle. This does not mean you have to join a health club or run a marathon every weekend. It means simply doing more physical things in your life. Walk to the store instead of driving, for example. This is not only better for you, but is cheaper as well. Mow the lawn, paint a room in your house, weed the garden, paint the whole house, go hiking or swimming (an excellent form of overall exercise), but *do something,* don't just sit there. Our bodies were built to be used and will function better and maintain longer if they are not allowed to atrophy and become rusty.

For those times when you must be seated (and it would be difficult to go very far through life — or even a day — without sitting), you have several options. You may invest in an ergonomically designed chair which adjusts to exactly to what your body needs. These are quite expensive, however, and are not necessarily within the reach of everyone's budget. You can use a small pillow or rolled-up towel behind your back. These are certainly not expensive, but can be very elusive — they shift every time you do and can actually end up causing discomfort. Or you can invest a few dollars to obtain one of the products designed to provide support in chairs and seats. The advantage of these units is that they are not too expensive and may be used in the home, the office or vehicle. Many people without back problems use such appliances simply because of the added comfort. And for those with back pain, their use can be invaluable.

One company which has supplied such products for

Back Supports

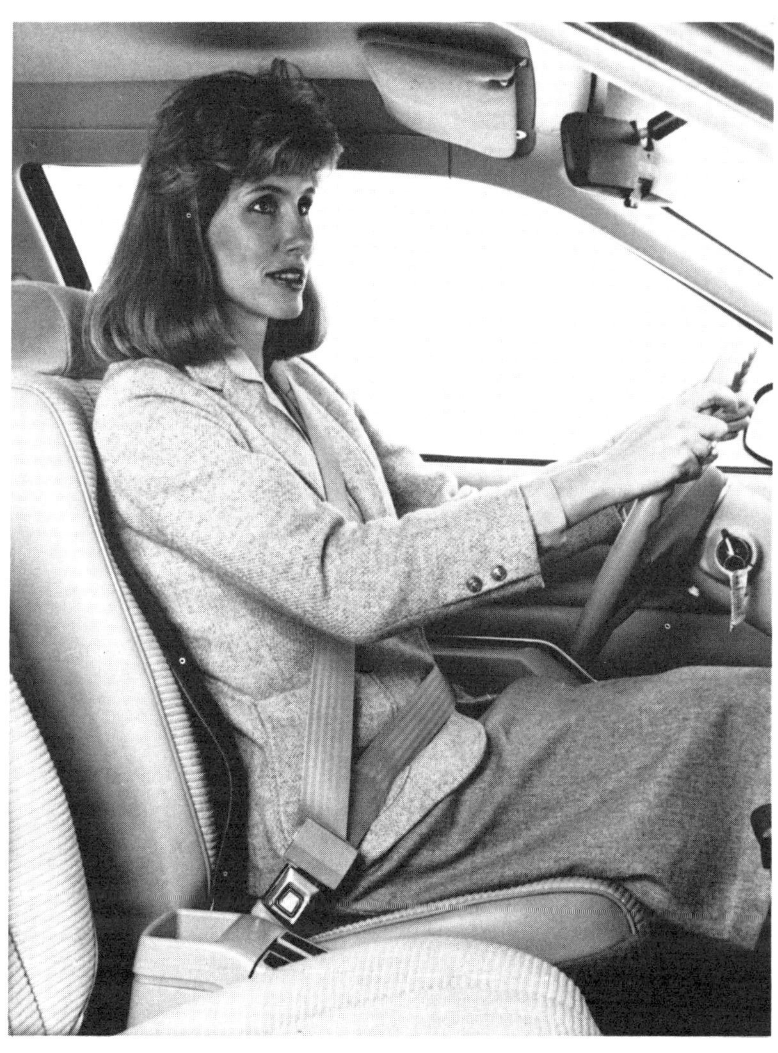

One of the most common usages of back support units is while operating a vehicle because of the added strain of bumping. People who spend much time driving or riding often find great relief from the support of such a unit. (Photo courtesy of McCarty's Sacro-Ease.)

over 45 years is McCarty's Sacro Ease® out of Idaho. They offer a wide range of seats, back units and lumbar pads to fit almost any need. They have too many models, in fact, to try to mention all of them here, so I will cover just a couple of their most popular models.

The Mini-Rest (MR) consists of a back portion with an attached lumbar pad which can be adjusted to provide support where needed. The retail price of this unit is $49. (All prices mentioned are, of course, only as of the time of this writing and are subject to change.)

The model BRS has the same features of the MR and also includes an attached seat for firm hip support in soft chairs. It sells for $78. Both units are also available in orthopedic models which do not include the lumbar pads but instead have bendable backs. These backs are custom fitted by dealers to shape to what the buyer needs.

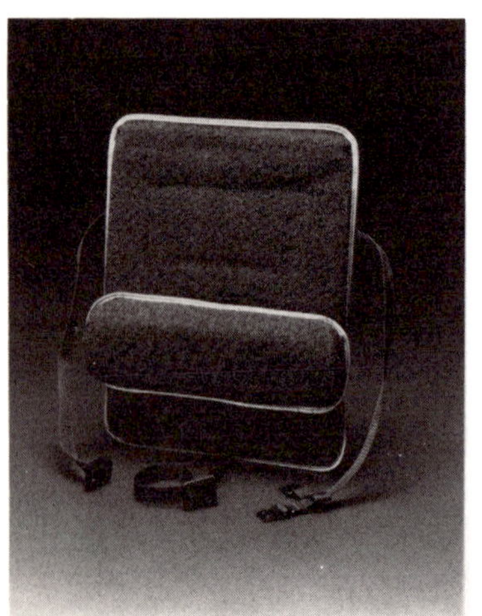 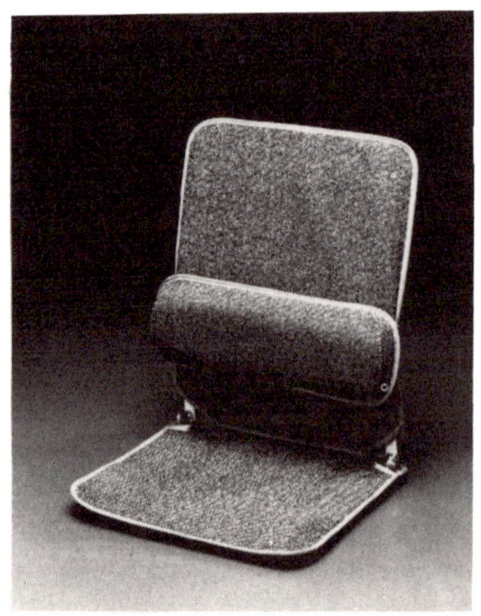

A couple of the most popular McCarty's Sacro-Ease lower back supports are the MINI-REST (left) and the Model BRS (right). Note the attached lumbar pads. These pads are adjustable for fitting the individuals's back. (Photos courtesy of McCarty's Sacro-Ease)

Since all Sacro Ease products are built with ⅛ inch carbon steel frames, the orthopedic models may be bent, straightened and rebent without fear of breaking. All of the cover fabrics are washable, too. I was also pleased to learn that all of their units include both a ten-day trial period and a five-year limited warranty. These units are for use with chairs and sofas as well as airplane and bus seats, cars, trucks and wheelchairs. And since they manufacture all their own products, if you happen to have an unusual sitting situation, they will be glad to give you a free estimate for designing a custom unit for your special needs.

When I spoke to the company president, Mr. William McCarty, he told me there are medical stores in all areas of the United States which carry Sacro-Ease products. If you can't find one near you or just want more information, contact McCarty's Sacro-Ease, 3329 Industrial Avenue, Coeur D'Alene, Idaho 83814. Better yet, save a stamp and call them toll free at 1-800-635-3557.

Another company which provides support units is Obus Forme® Ltd. of Toronto. Obus Forme is French for shell-shaped, and there is an interesting story behind the development of their back support unit.

The company president, Mr. Frank Roberts, was in a body cast for a period of time because of an arthritic back. When the cast was removed he cut it in half, added a layer of urethane foam to the half that fit his back, and put it in his car. The result was greater comfort while driving. The drawback was that it had to remain in the car because it weighed 50 pounds!

The shell of the Obus Forme back support is now made of a special polycarbonate instead of the original plaster, and the whole unit has been reduced to a svelte 32 ounces. It carries the BAC Seal of Approval and is being prescribed by doctors and hospitals in many countries. It has a non-allergenic covering (choice of colors) over a foam cushioning and sells for $69 in both the U.S. and Canada.

The cover and foam cushioning are expected to last three or four years before they need to be replaced, but the

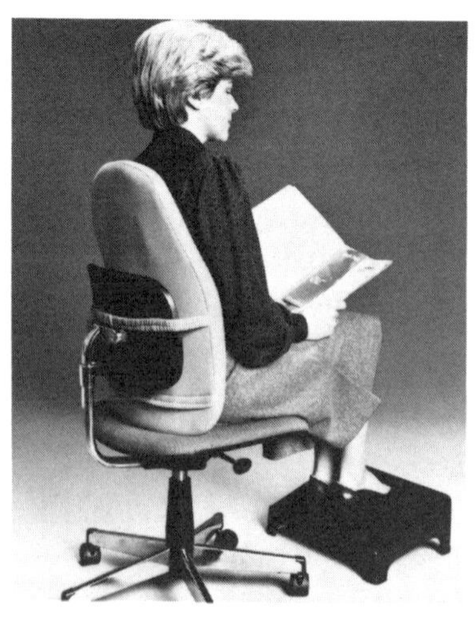 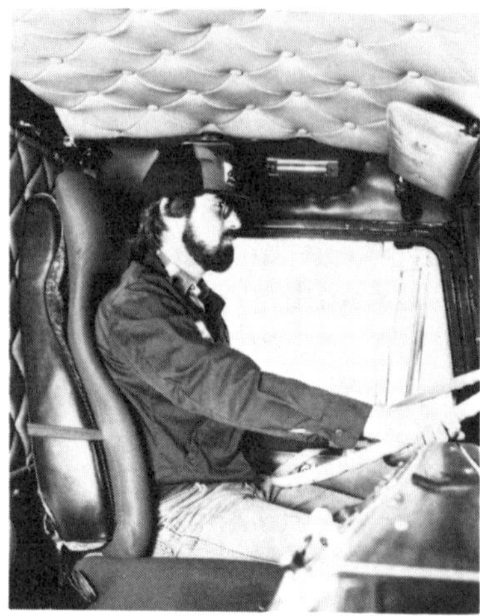

Back support units on the job. These are the Obus Forme Regular (left) and Hi Back (Right). (Photos courtesy of Obus Forme)

frame itself carries an unlimited warranty for the lifetime of the original purchaser.

Obus Forme also offers The SEAT for relief from sitting pressure. The SEAT may be used with or without the back support unit and is designed to distribute the upper body weight throughout the buttock region surrounding the ischial tuberosities or *sitting bones*. This reduces the stress that sitting places on the spine. It has an adjustable seat depth (a removable zip-out section) to allow for correct thigh support and may be folded up for easy carrying. The SEAT is also built around a moulded polycarbonate frame which carries a five-year guarantee. This unit sells for $49.

The Obus Forme Supporting Roll can be used for either lower back or neck support. It has a removable cover for cleaning and an elastic strap to hold it in position on a chair or car seat. It sells for $14.95.

Obus Forme products are available in medical stores and pharmacies in the United States and Canada. If you would like more information call the U.S. distributor, Camp, Int. toll free at 1-800-492-1088 or contact Obus Forme, Ltd. 550 Hopewell Avenue, Toronto, Ontario, Canada, M6E 2S6, telephone 416-785-1386.

None of the manufacturers I spoke to claimed that support units are the cure for back pain, and I agree with them. There simply is no substitute for good physical and emotional health when dealing with back problems. However, until the seating industry in general starts producing chairs and vehicle seats which maintain proper body alignment, back and hip support units can help a lot. For the healthy back they can make sitting more comfortable; for the troubled back they can help ease the pain and reduce further injury.

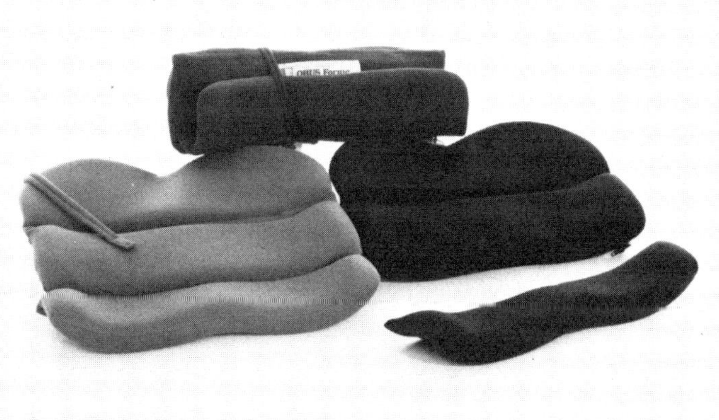

The Seat Buttock-Rest by Obus Forme. This picture shows three units: on the left is a complete unit, with the detachable section removed on the right. Upper-center shows The Seat folded for carrying. (Photos courtesy of Obus Forme)

So much of pain is emotional. If you wallow in self-pity, the pain gets worse. But, through joy and laughter, you can ease the anxiety and depression that are so often associated with chronic pain and thereby eliminate the suffering.

Alan D. Russakov, MD
Medical Director
Lourdes Regional Rehabilitation Center
Camden, New Jersey
The Complete Guide to Your Emotions & Your Health

Chapter 10

PATIENCE, JACKASS, PATIENCE

If you are one of the fortunate few who have the patience of a tree, this chapter will be of little use to you. If, on the other hand, like me, you have less patience than the average teenager, read on. We have found an element of your life which could use a little work.

Just as a good wine or compost pit requires time to properly age and ripen to its fullest potential, so does the healing process take time to be complete. One of the pitfalls of recuperation is attempting to resume full activities as soon as the pain is gone. Physicians have long complained about patients who discontinue medication once the symptoms disappear, even though the underlying cause of those symptoms may still be valid. A badly sprained ankle can take weeks to allow for pain-free walking, but it might be months before active usage may resume.

Back injuries are no different. After proper treatment has been obtained, it may still be some time before you want — or are able — to go back to normal activities. And the more you try to rush the recuperation process, the greater the risk of reinjury. Any exercise program — be it the limbering and stretching maneuvers while bedridden or the strengthening repetitions later — is meant to be built upon over a period of time. Try to stretch a muscle too fast or rush the healing process, and the piper may have to be paid.

I recently saw a sign hanging in a friend's office

which said, "Lord grant me patience, but I want it right now." We live in a time of fast food outlets, rush delivery service and instant mashed potatoes. We are able to fly from New York to Paris in just a few hours and have our film processed in one, but it still takes time to heal.

If you are currently healthy, wonderful. If you are presently limited to certain activities but still have mobility, fine. If you are now bedridden, miserable and lonely, rest assured I know what you are going through and have a few suggestions. Besides for the limbering and stretching exercises outlined elsewhere, here are a few ways you might pass your time.

1. Preliminary activities. These include all those little things you have meant to do for some time but, for one reason or another, have put off. They include taking an inventory of the holes, tiles, boards or swirls in your bedroom ceiling and cleaning the lint out of your navel. Admittedly these may not hold your attention for long, but they are at least an introduction to the fine art of killing time.

2. Watching television. There is enough pap in the average daily viewing schedule to make anyone forget their own problems. And if you concentrate on the soaps and detectives, you'll soon realize your current dilemma is minor compared to what's lying in wait for you *out there.*

3. Read books. *Thank you.* After you finish this one, I recommend you concentrate on peaceful and calming stories. The average bad back doesn't need the added stress of *The Exorcist.*

4. Talk to your spouse. You now are able to have those long, heart-to-heart talks you haven't seemed to have the time for lately. And who knows? You may come across the reason for your back pain.

5. Plan the perfect crime. This will provide hours and hours of fun and enjoyment. Be sure to cover all contingencies. Assume something will go wrong, determine what it may be, and devise a method to cover it. And don't

worry, even if you do come up with the perfect crime, you are in no condition to carry it out.

6. Write a book. I did, and apparently sold at least one copy. Don't feel badly if you don't know how to type. You are unable to sit up at a typewriter anyway. And if your book doesn't sell? Not to worry, we're just doing this to pass the time, remember?

7. Do a good *solve*. I must have done close to a zillion and a half crossword puzzles over the last 20 years. One word of caution, however. Be sure to work a puzzle in a book or magazine or at least use yesterday's paper. The frustration or not being able to come up with one or more of the words until tomorrow's paper isn't necessary right now.

8. Learn a language. There are plenty of good books and tapes on the market and at libraries for you to learn almost any foreign language you might want. Just make sure that in spite of your present state of mind, the language you pick up will be acceptable the next time you get back to the dinner table.

9. Enjoy an astral projection. Since the release of Shirley McLaine's *Out On A Limb,* many people are looking for out-of-body experiences. I have to admit I have not yet had the pleasure, but I will keep on trying. I would much rather visit the South of France and check out the latest in women's beach wear than stare at some dumb ceiling.

10. Fill in the blank. This one is up to you. The range of mental activities available is limited only by the imagination of the individual involved. It is a sad commentary when people with complete mental faculties and full physical mobility say "there's nothing to do." If prisoners of war in solitary confinement can make pets of spiders and do mathematical equations for months on end, it is obvious there is always something to do if only you are willing to look for it. If nothing else we can spend the time getting to know ourselves better, which might not be such a bad idea by itself.

    While some of the above suggestions may be just a bit

tongue-in-cheek, the reason for offering them is not. In order to insure a more complete recovery, allow the time for proper healing. If this entails counting the tiles in the ceiling or doing a crossword puzzle, so be it. You can save yourself a lot of further pain and aggravation by settling back, relaxing, and doing it right the first time.

Chapter 11

NEBC

I had a very refreshing experience recently when I walked into the New England Back Center in Burlington, Vermont. The Back Center is operated by University Orthopaedics of the University of Vermont and is located in an old school building separate from the hospital itself. My appointment was with Dr. Rowland Hazard, Medical Director of the Center, and one of the individuals responsible for its creation in the early part of 1986.

I have to admit that I entered the Center with a certain amount of trepedation based upon too many years of personal experience with doctors and their offices. To my surprise the waiting room was not filled with patients waiting for an appointment scheduled for over an hour ago. Nor was there any hint of that peculiar odor which says you must be sick, why else would you be here? As a matter of fact, the waiting room — I really should call it the reception room, for that's more what it is — was as bright and cheery as the receptionist herself. She seemed happy to see me even though she had no idea who I was or why I was there, and didn't make me feel as if I was interrupting her schedule by showing up at her desk unannounced. So far, so good.

Dr. Hazard made his appearance in a timely manner and continued the favorable impression. Even though I'm sure he has a very tight schedule himself, there was no sense of being rushed as he showed me around the facility and sat down with a cup of coffee to explain the operation and answer any questions I had.

The New England Back Center (NEBC) is a relatively new (very new to me) approach to the treatment of back problems. The patients they receive are not the ones who miss a few days work a year, but are people who, on the average, have been on medical disability for eleven months. They have been through medical evaluations and various treatments and still are unable to return to work or resume many of their previous activities. For many this could be seen as a "court of final appeal."

As we toured the exercise room, the machine room (for testing and evaluation of physical conditioning), the recreation room and other parts of the facility, I was surprised to still not detect any of the tell-tale *you are sick* signs. Dr. Hazard explained that the center stresses *wellness,* not *illness.* Individuals attending the three-week treatment stay at local hotels, not in one of the hospital rooms about a block away. They spend ten hours a day stretching, lifting, building endurance and participating in training sessions on relaxation techniques, biofeedback, job hunting and individual counseling. One of the keys to the program, according to Dr. Hazard, is that it "treats the whole person, not just the back. Chronic back pain affects people's moods, relationships, their work lives, and their self-esteem...its not just the back that gets out of shape."

The NEBC program is patterned after the PRIDE Institute, affiliated with the University of Texas in Dallas, and was developed by Dr. Tom Mayer. During a two-year study period the PRIDE Institute saw 80% of its patients returning to work, compared to the 20-30% from conventional treatment.

The program was brought to New England in part because of Dr. Hazard. As he explained to me, he had a private practice as an internist and realized there really wasn't much he could do for his patients complaining of back pain. After searching through the existing medical books on the subject, he found there just wasn't much

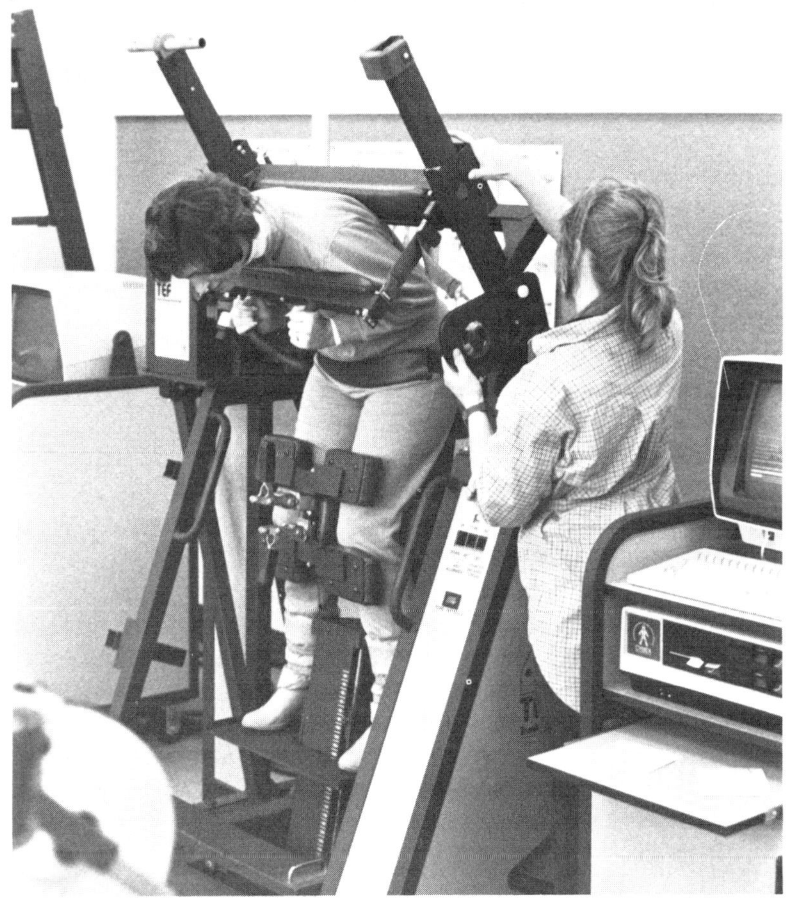

The Trunk Extension Flexion (T.E.F.), manufactured by Cybex, is used to test the stomach (flexion) and back (extension) strength of individuals at the New England Back Center. The computer and monitor at the right of the photograph are used to chart the findings of the tests over a period of time. Here we see Linda Harvey, R.P.T. demonstrate the use of the T.E.F. by running Karen through the paces. Although the machine is intimidating in appearance, Karen assured me it was actually quite painless.

information available and began looking elsewhere for help with his back patients. Upon examination of two or three programs being offered around the world, the PRIDE Institute's was the one chosen because of its demonstrated effectiveness.

On my second visit to the Back Center I was accompanied by my wife, Karen, who was to serve as a model for some photographs of the equipment. We met with the administrator, Ken Yates, who continued the feeling of friendly assistance I had encountered on my first visit. He

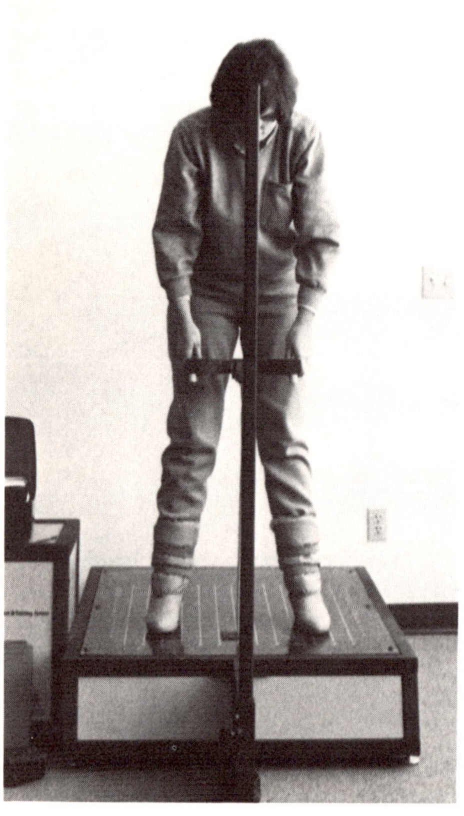

Another machine employed by the Back Center is the Liftask, also manufactured by Cybex. This is used to test the lifting capabilities of individuals before entering the center, and again after completion of the program to demonstrate increased strength.

introduced us to Linda Harvey and Sheila Reid, registered physical therapists, who demonstrated the various machines used for the physical evaluation of patients. Patients are tested both upon entering the center and again as they leave, with periodic follow ups after release. As it was explained to us, a proper balance of strength should show the back (extension) about 25% higher than the stomach (flexion). The chart readings give the person a chance to see where their physical weaknesses lie and to follow their improvement from the program.

After our visit to the physical therapy section, Ken Yates took us to the psychology department. There we met the staff psychologist, Steve Kalisch, PhD and his two personable clinical psychology interns, Nancy Silberg and Ava Melion. Steve, as he is called around the center, discussed the emotional and environmental influences in back problems.

As I have mentioned, a person's response to injury and pain may be greatly complicated by fear of the pain itself or of the feeling of being unable to perform ordinary functions. The stresses of the individual's life may also enter the picture. If we are *uptight* (and I use the word intentionally) about elements of our domestic or employment situation, for example, we may easily transfer much of that tension into parts of our body. Necks and backs are the classic recipients of such transferral. And if there is already an existing injury in the area, the focus of muscle constriction can easily increase the severity or lengthen the duration of the episode.

To give us a visible demonstration of the value of relaxation, Steve put Karen on the biofeedback machine. This was my first exposure to such an instrument and I found it most fascinating. Connections are made by the placement of small suction cups on the forehead. It seems that the muscles just above the eye are great indicators of tension in the body. The impulses are then relayed to a monitor, which is a small television-type screen and contains a series of multicolored columns. The color of the columns indicates the degree of tension experienced. High anxiety is reflected by a predominance of orange, with yellow, light blue and dark blue showing a progression into deep relaxation. This gives the individual the chance to actually monitor their emotional state as it changes.

As Steve said would probably be the case, Karen's first reading was almost solid orange. By consciously trying to relax her body she was able to bring about a little more yellow, but that was about it. Even though she was seated in a large, comfortable chair and in a room cut off from distractions, she was unable to lower herself into the more relaxed state indicated by the light and dark blue columns. This is a very common response, according to Steve, given the stressful lives most of us lead. And if we happen to be experiencing pain at the time, relaxation is even more difficult — and yet more necessary — to attain.

To assist her, Steve then played an audio relaxation tape for Karen. These are designed to gently talk a person down from the anxiety they are experiencing, to a deeper, healthier state of relaxation.

As the minutes passed, the screen developed more yellow and a little of the light blue as Karen was beginning to let go of her apprehension. Soon a little of the dark blue made its appearance and we knew the tape was working. When it was time for the session to end, I had to practically haul my Raggedy Ann wife up from her easy chair. On our trip home from the Back Center that afternoon, Karen was the most relaxed I have seen her in some time.

This same technique can be used in the privacy of your own home. Without the monitor, of course. Designate a period of time during the day which is just for you. Hang a Do Not Disturb sign on the door and take the phone off the hook, if necessary, but make it a period free of distractions if at all possible. Dim the lights or pull the shades and nestle yourself into a nice soft easy chair or sofa which fits and supports you well. Then just let yourself go. Free your mind of distracting thoughts and worries and allow all the muscles in your body to loosen. For this period of time you don't

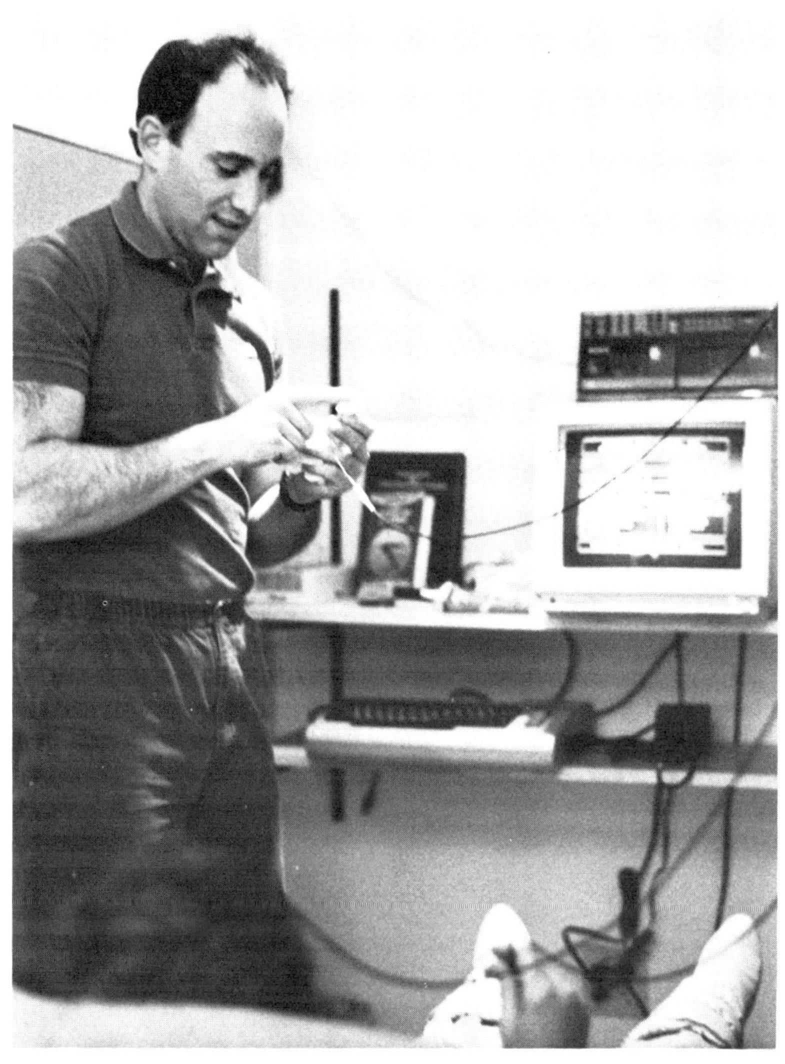

Steve Kalisch, PhD prepares Karen for the biofeedback machine demonstration. At the right of the photograph is the monitor which displays the state of tension or relaxation of the user. On top of the monitor is the tape player for the relaxation tapes which are an integral part of this experience.

have to pay any bills or get the kids through college. You don't even have to talk to your boss about that problem on the job right now. Just relax and let it go. You might be surprised to see how much better you feel after a while.

A little soft music playing quietly in the background can help during these times as well. Better yet, use one of the relaxation tapes to help you, at least while you are learning to truly relax. The tape Steve has found to be one of the best is part of a series including Progressive Relaxation and Deep Muscle Relaxation, and is available from Stress Man-

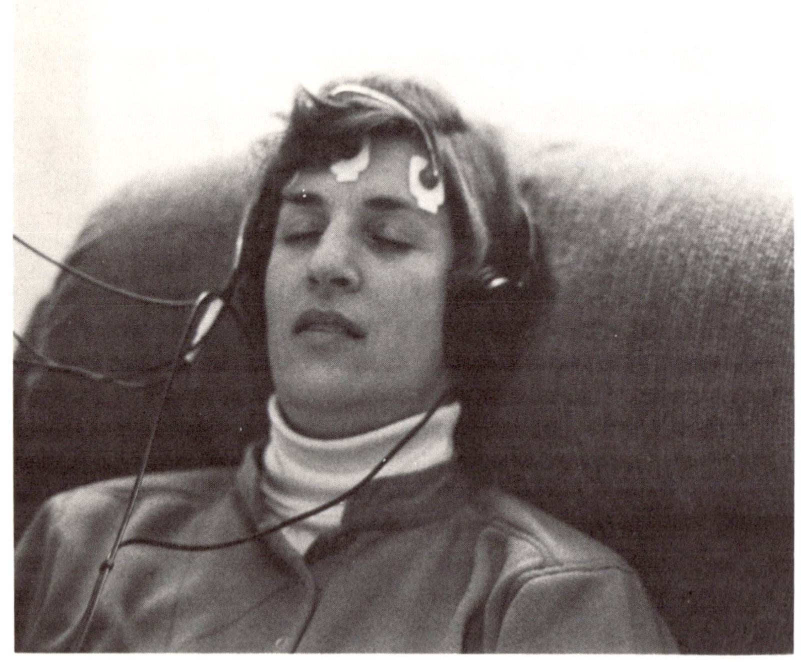

Karen relaxing on the biofeedback machine. Note the large, soft recliner in which she is seated for extra comfort. Ordinarily the lights would be dimmed as well, to reduce any outside distractions. In this photograph Karen is wearing headphones for listening to the relaxation tape, although Steve indicated that usually people find them more distracting and prefer to listen to the tape in the open room.

agement Research Associates, Inc., PO Box 2232, Houston, TX 77251.

Another good relaxation tape is available from Bannister Publications for $11.95 ($1.00 S&H). Write to them at Box 63, Port Henry, NY 12974 and tell them you would like a copy of their relaxation tape sent right away. Since they are also the publishers of this book, I'm sure they will want to accommodate their readers. But whatever technique or method you use, please keep in mind that true relaxation is an important element in maintaining a healthy, balanced life. It reduces damaging stress and tension, gives the body a chance to recuperate, and generally helps put our lives back into proper perspective. And the best part is you don't even have to work at it — just let go and enjoy.

Because of its short time in operation, the overall effectiveness of the New England Back Center remains to be proven. As one who has had considerable personal experience with a bad back, however, everything I saw and heard there made an awful lot of sense to me. They seem to be on the right track in their approach to back problems, something which has been needed for a long time. And if the cheerful attitudes and sincerity of the individuals involved are any measure, I suspect they will be a great help to many people.

You may contact the New England Back Center at 38 Fletcher Place, Burlington, VT 05401 or call them at 802-656-4680.

Chapter 12

FOR WOMEN ONLY

Even in these days of equal rights and parity between the sexes, there are a few elements of back pain which are unique to women. Granted this creates an inequality between the sexes, but whether men should be upset because they are left out or women should feel the offended party because of extra crosses to bear is a moot point and one I certainly don't want to get into here. The fact of the matter is differences *do* exist, and being aware of them may help your situation.

First of all, women's bodies were not designed to lift heavy weights. And yet it is women who carry Junior not only through the term of their pregnancy, but often too far into his growing process as well. Babies have to be carried for awhile, granted, but lugging the little darling around when he is old enough to outrun you is only asking for trouble. Even when he is still young enough to be lifted out of a crib, be careful how it is done. Any lifting which has to be performed is best done by first bringing the object close to your body and then lifting with the legs as well as the back. Having to lean over the jail-cell bars of the crib and lifting with your arms out in front is going to create a strain you really don't need. If at all possible lower the crib wall first, pull your blessed bundle to you, and then stand up. You'll appreciate it in the long run.

Pregnancy itself is a classic cause of backaches.

There is not only the standard problem of a weight being carried in front of the body which puts an extra strain on the back for support, but there is the added complication of the loosening process of the pelvic ligaments to allow for the birth. This is a natural and necessary process which will usually correct itself automatically following delivery. In the meantime, however, you have a situation which could use the assistance of healthy muscles to help keep things in order. Check with your obstetrician or hospital for recommended exercises which may be performed throughout the course of pregnancy. These will help you avoid some of the customary aches and pains associated with this process and may make your delivery easier as well.

Surprisingly enough, breasts can be a source of back pain in women, both directly and indirectly. Large, pendulous breasts, especially on a slight-framed woman, can generate the same problem as that of pregnancy or the carrying of any weight in front of your body. Extra strain is placed on the back to maintain proper body alignment. In extreme cases surgery can be performed to reduce the size of the breasts. In most cases, however, wearing a specially designed, more supportive bra will help.

A less direct but equally effective contributor to back pain for women comes from the other end of the spectrum — the tiny, budding breasts of young girls. Puberty is usually a complicated process at best. We are on our way out of the carefree stage of childhood and on our way into the more complex and unknown world of adults. Our attitudes and emotions begin to shift subtly in ways we don't always understand and life becomes exciting and a little scary. And then our bodies start doing things, too. In young girls, the rosebud nipples are about the first outward sign to the world that changes are taking place. Some girls find this embarrassing and involuntarily round their shoulders forward to hide the evidence. Occasionally this will follow on into a life pattern of bad posture which will have to be answered for down the line. I'm afraid I don't have a good answer for this one — I've tried talking to my own teenagers too many times to pretend that they will change bad habits simply at our suggestion. (I'm sure glad my parents never had to deal with a hard-headed teenager.) But if we are able to somehow correct this particular situation if it develops, this is at least one problem our children will be able to avoid in years to come.

Other factors which contribute to back pain in women are internal and not nearly as obvious. Menstruation will sometimes cause back pain of its own accord. At other times it can aggravate an already existing back pain. Infections of the ovaries or fallopian tubes may refer pain to the back. A tipped uterus can create a pull to the attached ligaments and generate one whale of a backache. I have already mentioned the story of the woman I knew who suffered from backaches for a long time before the problem of a tipped uterus was discovered. The vaginal insertion of a frame to support and realign her uterus stopped the pain almost immediately.

These examples once again point out the oft' repeated refrain — proper diagnosis is essential for proper treatment. The key to back pain is to treat the *cause*, not the symptom.

Chapter 13

TRICKS OF THE *TRADE*

Anyone suffering from back problems long enough will learn a few things they can — and cannot — do to make life more comfortable. Here are a few simple suggestions which I have found to help.

DO'S

1. Maintain good posture. Besides for appearing that life has already gotten the better of you, sloppy posture is an invitation for future problems in your back.
2. Maintain a regular program of back exercises. Don't worry, we're not talking strain and pain here. We're talking stretching and limbering movements which help keep things where they belong. Even if you happen to be a loyal member of The Society of Sweat and Hurt and are working on building the body beautiful, keep in mind that bountiful biceps won't compensate for a sacro spasm. These maneuvers are not nearly as dramatic as curling 200 pounds or bench pressing a horse, but they may be done at home (in bed, even) and will help keep your back healthier. (See Chapter 6, Exercise)
3. Try moist heat when using a heating pad. This can be done by simply placing a wet, warm washcloth between the heating pad and your body. Of course, you want to make sure your heating pad has a rubber or plastic covering. The value of shock treatment

through shorting out a heating pad leaves a lot to be desired. I had it happen once and didn't like it at all.

4. Speaking of heating pads (or hot water bottles), if you are applying heat, keep the duration short, usually 10 to 15 minutes, and make sure its not too hot. A little heat can relax muscles and increase circulation to aid healing, but too much heat for too long will create swelling, which is counterproductive.

5. Keep your weight within reasonable limits. The secret to many back problems is simply misalignment of bones, muscles or ligaments. Carrying a potbelly is no different than carrying any weight out in front of your body—it forces the musculature of your back to overcompensate to maintain a proper center of gravity. It has recently been determined that overweight people who carry their fat in the belly are more prone to heart problems than people whose fat is more evenly distributed in their hips and thighs. Potbellies don't do anything to help back problems, either.

6. If your bedroom is on the second floor, have someone set up a bed downstairs for you for those times when mobility is almost nil. If not the whole bed, just having a mattress dragged down the stairs to put on the living room floor will help. As with most of life's little lessons, I learned this one the hard way. Near the end of one three-week episode I thought I felt well enough to go downstairs for lunch one afternoon. I was tired of bed and wanted to be with the family for a change. Halfway through lunch my back began tightening and I tried to make it back upstairs to bed. By the sixth stair I was crawling on my hands and knees and crying like a baby. Without going into the rest of the gory details, suffice it to say the fewer steps you have to climb when your back is out, the better off you will be.

7. This next suggestion may seem too basic to even mention, but mention it I will because it has been the

source of many an unpleasant surprise. While doing almost anything, make slow, deliberate movements. Sudden twists or turns, jerky lifting or bending (and I use the term *jerky* deliberately), will often reward the individual with a prolonged vacation in bed. I have changed what seems like three million flat tires in my lifetime with nothing more to show for it than dirty hands. One time, however, I was in a hurry and lifted and pushed the tire out in front without first balancing my position. And away we went. The two seconds I tried to save by not first adjusting my stance cost me three days. If you think that was a good return on my investment, I have this nifty little bridge you might be interested in buying.

8. While lying in bed on your back, try a pillow under your knees. Straight legs can sometimes add an extra strain or pull to your lower back. On your side, its usually more comfortable to have one or both knees bent, and placing a pillow between your knees can help maintain better body alignment. A pillow under your head usually helps when lying on your side, but is often worse when on your back. One of the keys during back episodes is *if it feels good, do it.* When you find a comfortable position, enjoy it, because it means that your muscles are able to relax at least a little more and are therefore able to proceed with the healing process.

9. This is the most important of the *DO'S* and really should be in the number one position, but I have always liked to save the best for last. When you experience a back injury, get help ASAP. The longer you put off seeing a health-care practitioner, the more likely the problem will be further aggravated, and therefore take longer to recuperate. I cover complications several places in the book so I will not beat those same dead horses here. For now, just accept that the sooner you receive treatment, the better off you will be.

DON'TS

1. Don't push it too far. This goes hand-in-glove with the last *DO* and is probably the most difficult lesson I had to learn in dealing with a bad back. I like doing things and I hate to be confined. As a result I have many times tried to bull my way through a situation when I should have stayed in bed and healed first. What I usually received for my efforts was an extended stay in bed. I'm not saying to climb into bed every time a minor ache or pain is experienced. This can be counterproductive. What I am talking about are those times when damage has been done and correction or healing is necessary.

2. In the same vein, if seeing someone at home is easier than going out when your back is painful, then don't go out. If staying in bed hurts less than getting up, don't get up. You might be surprised at what may be accomplished without having to further aggravate your back.

While it is true that healing takes place better in a more relaxed atmosphere, and that extra stresses and tensions are best avoided if possible, many obligations may still be met if the situation demands it. I have conducted business meetings in person and on the telephone, played card games with friends and, in general, carried on the almost normal routine of a regular day while stationed on my mattress on the living room floor. While I admit this is not the optimum scenario for business and social interaction, it beats going broke or being lonely.

3. Don't wear belts which are too tight. Besides being unattractive on most individuals, a tight belt can serve the same function as a tourniquet applied to an arm or leg.

4. Don't sit on a fat wallet. Even though some of us seldom have the opportunity for such a problem, it is something of which you should be aware. Having one's rear end partially placed on a bundle of bucks

and credit cards will elevate one hip to the detriment of the other. Again, alignment.

5. Don't use combinations of heat treatments at the same time. The application of heat (not too hot and not too long) can sometimes help a sore spot by increasing the circulation of blood to the area and relaxing the muscles. However, this is another case of *if a little is good, at lot t'aint necessarily better.* I once had my wife apply a liberal portion of *Heet* to my back before climbing into a hot bathtub to relax. It was a blistering experience.

6. Don't bend or lift from your waist. We were provided knees for more than just proposing or groveling. Bending and lifting are a couple of good times to use them.

7. Don't ride in a car or sit in a chair any more than absolutely necessary when your back is painful. Sitting is about the worst position for backs. If you *must* sit up for whatever reason, use a pillow or supporting device to fill in that empty space between your lower back and the seat. (See Chapter 10, Back Supports).

8. Don't settle for one opinion, especially if the recommended treatment doesn't help much. There are a variety of reasons for back pain, some more involved than others, and they are often difficult to diagnose.

9. Don't accept treatment from unqualified individuals. This may seem rather basic, but I've seen people who had friends pop their neck, twist their legs and torsos and even walk on their back. It gives me the shivers. If you won't at least see practitioners who are qualified to try to find the problem, then give the Boston Strangler a call. Guaranteed you won't feel any pain when he is finished with his treatment.

10. Don't jump on trampolines, don't play NFL football and don't ride rodeo bulls. Okay, my tongue just slipped into my cheek, again. What I'm saying is be reasonable as to what you do while experiencing

back problems. When all is said and done, there's really no substitute for common sense.

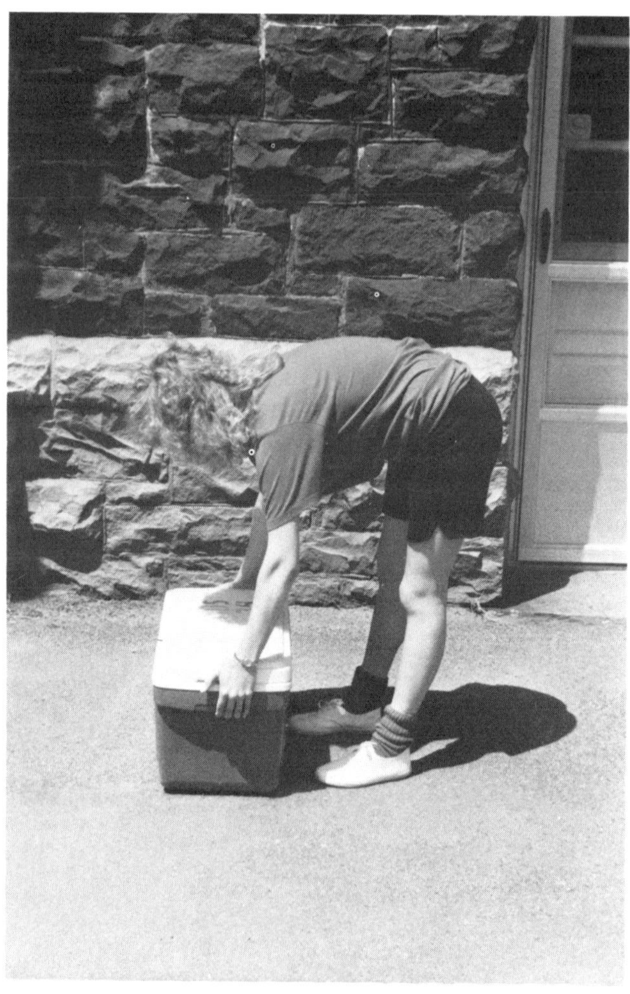

INCORRECT. This is a natural tendency for many people—especially in advancing years as the legs start to go—but is a dangerous position for the back. Note the leverage involved—the majority of the lift and pull is centered directly in the small of the back.

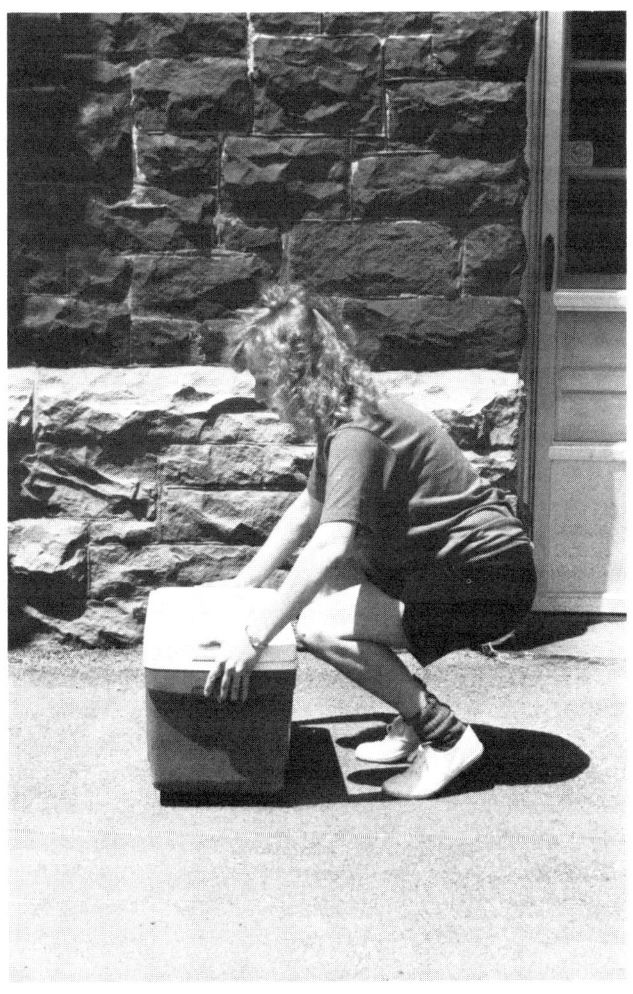

CORRECT. *Placing the object closer to the body and distributing the weight between back and leg muscles is much safer and more sightly for the casual observer.*

...over the years I have encountered a surprising number of instances in which, to all appearances, patients have laughed themselves back to health...

Raymond A. Moody, Jr., MD
Laugh after Laugh: The Healing Power of Humor

Chapter 14

MAKING YOUR LIFE WORK

This may well become the most controversial chapter in the book, but in my opinion no comprehensive treatment of back problems would be complete without it. In this chapter we will be looking at many areas of our lives: psychology, philosophy, work patterns, social structures, relationships, beliefs, aspirations and attitudes. In short, almost every aspect of life except back pain...directly. And yet these elements are all part of the overall framework in which we live (survive), work (struggle) and play (escape), and in which there is an increasingly high incidence of back pain, along with chemical abuse, emotional disturbance and suicide. When viewed in this light it becomes apparent that many lives are not *working*.

Why should this be?

There is a story of a young prince in a mythical kingdom which I find quite interesting. This young man was handsome, wealthy, born of royal blood, enjoyed good health and the respect and admiration of all the people in the kingdom and was to have his choice of the village virgins when it came time to marry. Everyone knew he was destined to live happily ever after.

And no one understood why he took his own life in the prime of his years.

Why would he do such a thing? In the current vernacular he *had it made*. He enjoyed all the aspects of life the townsfolk were working so hard to attain: money, fame, power and admiration. Why should he kill himself and throw all that away?

Perhaps it was because he was simply living out a role written for him long before he was born. His life consisted of doing what was *expected* of him; of living out what the villagers *thought* were their own goals and dreams, with little or no allowance for being or doing what *he* wanted to be or do. Set up on this throne, as it were, he would never be able to experience the true feelings of friendship and community which were taken for granted by the townsfolk, and the emotion of love for him would always be tainted by his position. He would simply never have been allowed to live out a *normal* life, a life of his own choosing.

What does this mean to us?

EXPECTATIONS

Most of our lives are spent fulfilling (or trying to fulfill) the expectations of others. As little children we are expected to be quiet and tidy and not bother the adults. When we get to school we are expected to study hard and get the grades necessary to prepare for the college we are expected to attend, where the same rules apply in preparing for the balance of our lives. The relationships we establish along the way are rife with expected codes of behavior, and when we enter the work force the expectations really pile up. There is very little action within a job environment which is free of expected behavior. Either we do what is expected of us on the job or we are out on our ear, and since we are expected to support ourselves and our families...well, we have just traveled full circle, haven't we?

Beneath all these everyday expectations lie the biggies which are offered by society (and television) and accepted by us: that we will be *successful* in terms of wealth, fame and power. (For some individuals these life expectations are reversed — that they will *not* be successful, that they are in fact *born to lose*. This can be even more damaging, but is another consideration entirely and will not be addressed at this time.)

I'm sure you have seen — if not lived through — the portrayal of these *positive* expectations: the young buck who feels he has the answers to all of life's questions and who *knows* he will go on to do great things. And many do. Many others, however, find themselves a few years down the road slogging along in a job they don't enjoy, but one they feel locked into as they struggle to keep up with the constant flow of monthly bills. And soon they begin to wonder where the magic went.

They have accepted the socially defined expectations of success, yet somehow have not quite been able to get there. The initial feelings of disappointment and frustration can easily evolve into *inability* and *failure*. These strugglers may in fact have a wonderful family structure and the support and love of many people, but still cannot accept themselves as worthy due to their perceived failure, and often find excuses and escapes in the form of chemical abuse, emotional disturbance, a myriad of physical ailments and, occasionally, suicide.

But what of those individuals who "make it?"

ITS LONELY AT THE TOP

For those who go on to become socially accepted successes — captains of industry, world and government leaders, *stars,* public figures and controllers of wealth and power—there is an old adage which claims that *its lonely at the top.* For many of us looking up (such as the villagers), this may be difficult to accept. After all, don't they have everything we are working so hard to achieve? And yet there is often a price which must be paid to achieve these positions. This price can include the loss of close family ties due to demanding work schedules, the lack of the friendships and comaraderie otherwise found in the work place and the absence of love without motivation. Imagine the feeling of never being quite sure whether the affections offered are for you or for some possible gain or advancement on the part of the offerer.

These *winners* may have all the wealth and power they want (although sometimes no amount is ever enough), but without the close personal ties of humanity may still perceive themselves as unworthy and find excuses and escapes from their situation. These can include chemical abuse, emotional disturbance, a myriad of physical ailments and, occasionally, suicide. Sounds familiar, doesn't it?

Is this saying, then, that there is no reason to go on? That whether we *make it* or not we are still destined for unhappiness?

Absolutely not! The purpose of this chapter is to find ways to make our lives work; to be able to experience the joy of living regardless of social standing or income level; to enable ourselves to live without the excuses and escapes so often deemed necessary; to learn to accept ourselves *as we are.*

There is a Jimmy Stewart movie about a six-foot rabbit named (and entitled) Harvey which I would highly recommend to anyone who has not seen it at least two or three times. It is not only enjoyable, but has quite a message as well. Jimmy Stewart plays the role of a rather eccentric gentleman by the name of Elwood P. Dowd, to whom Harvey is a close confidant. I use the term *eccentric* as defined by social standards because Elwood does not accept the stresses and tensions in his life which society seems to expect of its citizens. He rolls with the punches and *experiences* his surroundings rather than going into conflict with them.

At one point in the film Elwood is conversing with a psychiatrist who, as the rest of the cast, is as yet unable to *see* Harvey. The doctor has asked Elwood why he is not upset about certain dramatic events which have just taken place in the story line and Elwood replies, "I just enjoy being wherever I am, doing whatever I am doing." Sounds simple, doesn't it?

K.I.S.S.

My father has said for many years, "Don't take life too seriously, you won't get out of it alive, anyway." This statement has nothing to do with theology or life-after-death or the existence or absence of reincarnational recycling. It deals strictly with the manner in which we handle the everyday involvements in our lives. Too often we build huge mountains out of the molehills of our existence and — to place yet another float in this parade of cliches — stir up tremendous tempests in our daily teapots. Granted some of this activity is to stimulate what we may see as an otherwise mundane existence, but too often it is carried to a point of unnecessary stress and tension.

Another way of stating this idea is K.I.S.S. (Keep It Simple, Stupid). If you need to take offense to this, go ahead, but it is not meant to offend. It is meant to point out what so many of us do to ourselves. We often complicate our lives to the point of near impossibility by the acceptance of unnecessary responsibility and expectation, needless worry and concern. As *responsible* adults we have sufficient cares and concerns to last a lifetime, and which should be addressed and handled. Where a change can take place is in accepting those which are *real* and rejecting those which are unnecessary. Sometimes it takes a pretty close look to tell the difference, but it can be well worth the time.

Our lives are full of *stuff* which we consider good or bad, wanted or unwanted, positive or negative. We feel we have a fairly clear grasp of right and wrong and of what we want and don't want. And yet history shows us repeatedly that what may be deemed desirable at one point in time may turn out to be undesirable at another; that an unwanted occurrence may be beneficial in the long run. An employee will be unhappy, for example, when he is laid off from even a mediocre job. But when he then finds another which has better working conditions and pays more to boot, he will accept the change as *good.*

This is not to say that we should all sit back and let the world *happen to us*. Our *real* responsibility as individuals is to learn to discern what is meaningful and what is not; to prioritize our lives and focus on the true and discard the false. Continually jousting phony windmills and arguing unnecessary issues can lead to frustration, anger and despair; can develop a life which is not working.

Where do we find the power or ability to know what is truly meaningful?

IF YOU WANT A JOB DONE RIGHT...

There are many sources of assistance available to us for dealing with certain areas of our lives — our pastor, priest, rabbi, spiritual leader, psychologist, psychiatrist, psychoanalyst, counselor, friends, family, bartender. They all listen to our problems, make suggestions and offer advice, but when push comes down to shove it is ultimately the individual involved who makes the decision as to a course of action for himself. And this is as it should be. If we claim *my friend said I should quit this job* or *my counselor told me to get a divorce,* we are copping out; we are avoiding the responsibility for our own lives and trying to place the blame on others. Not only is this unfair to the other party, it just won't wash. If we are unwilling to accept responsibility for our own lives, why should we expect someone else to? *How* can we expect someone else to?

YES, BUT...

In psychology we are told that we hold on to certain problems because they satisfy some underlying need in our lives. This is not always easy to understand. Why should someone retain a feeling of inability if the rest of the world perceives them as capable, for example, or why would anyone accept a physical disability that wasn't *real?* The answers to these questions are many and varied and not always easy to discover, but the fact remains that they do happen, they are done. And more often than we might expect. And, until the underlying cause is addressed and rectified, there will be a devil of a time trying to change the symptom.

I'm sure you have had the experience of a friend coming to you with a *problem* to be resolved, the resolution to which turned out to be seemingly impossible. It could be something as simple as getting to a nearby town for a meeting he feels he is expected to attend, but his car is on the blink. You suggest that he might have the car repaired and his response is "yes, but...it would take too long." You then offer the idea of his borrowing someone else's car and he replies, "yes, but...I don't like the responsibility of doing that." You then try the taking of a cab, "yes, but...that would cost too much." Okay, how about taking a bus? "Yes, but...then I wouldn't have any way of getting home after the busses quit running."

It usually doesn't take long to realize that you could offer suggestions all day and it wouldn't help. You are only covering the symptom problems when the real trouble is that your friend doesn't want to go the meeting. He feels he *should* go because it is expected of him, but he *really doesn't want to go!* By his rationalizing the situation in this manner he will feel that he has made the attempt to go, just couldn't get there, that's all. In time, he may even feel that he probably *did* want to go, its just that the circumstances were beyond his control. The unfortunate aspect of this example is that the only one he's fooling, ultimately, is himself. And the larger the arena of expectation in which this game is played, the more damaging — to the self — it becomes.

This game is often played against the expectations placed upon us by others, but may also be played to defeat our own hopes and dreams, usually out of fear. *Well, sure, I'd like to go back to school and become a doctor, but...I can't just quit my job* (I might not make it through medical school and then where would I be?); *I'd really like to have children, but...we can't afford them right now* (I'm afraid of the responsibility); *I would like to act on the stage, but...I don't have time for all the rehearsals* (I'm scared witless); *I would like to be a writer, but...I have too many things to do as it is* (What if nobody liked my books?). And the more this game is played, the stronger will become the feeling of inadequacy and the more the game needs to be played for protection. This can continue in an ever increasing cycle to the point of social and individual paralysis.

How, then, can we break this vicious cycle of self-destruction?

TRUTH, JUSTICE AND THE AMERICAN WAY

Since we are not Superman, most of us don't have complete control over Justice and The American Way, but we do have absolute control over Truth, at least as it applies to ourselves. If the friend in the first example had been honest with himself — the meeting was going to be boring, he already knew the material to be covered and, besides, watching Monday Night Football would be much more enjoyable — he would not only have saved a lot of your time and his, but would probably have a higher opinion of himself as well. Its difficult to lie to yourself and expect to get away with it completely. There is almost always that damned niggling little voice that says *I heard what you said. You know better than that.* And the trouble is, you *do* know better than that.

As for rationalizing away dreams out of fear, again, truth can be the key.

If your dream is to be the actor, for example, but you have rationalized to yourself that you can't do it because you don't have time for all the rehearsals, rest assured you will find plenty of *commitments* in your life to prevent you from ever going on stage. You have built a phony obstacle for yourself and will be very glad to reinforce it. If, on the other hand, you identify the truth of the matter — that you are frightened silly of getting up in front of all those people — you will be able to at least deal with the root issue. Fear can often be overcome or at least managed. I don't know of any performers who weren't frightened their first few times on stage. That's part of the thrill. Some experience intense fear every time they appear, but they still go on. They don't accept any excuses to prevent their doing what they really want to do.

Now that we have started being honest with ourselves, let's expand outward to dealing truthfully with others.

OH, WHAT A TANGLED WEB WE WEAVE...

My wife is a good cook. Everything she prepares is done well. Occasionally, however, she uses a *recipe* which I don't enjoy. But it took me a long time to learn the difference.

When we were first married she fixed a meal which contained an ingredient which didn't agree with me. When she asked how it was, I replied "its fine." I didn't think I was lying, exactly, maybe stretching the truth a little, but I didn't want to hurt her feelings. The punishment for my misrepresentation, however, was visited upon me — or served to me — several times over the next few years. I finally realized I could tell her I didn't enjoy that particular dish without saying that she was a bad cook. That opened a lot of doors in our lives and has led to more truthful communications in our marriage.

Child psychologists point out the difference in chastising a child by telling him he is a *bad boy* as compared to saying we don't like what he *did,* but we still like *him.* And there is a major difference. A child who has erred but is still loved has a chance to correct what he is doing. A *bad boy,* on the other hand, may live with that identity for a long time.

A very common form of harmful — although well-intentioned — communications is what I call Spy Vs Spy.

This is where we tell someone what we *think* they want to hear, regardless of our true feelings on the matter. You know the situation: John and Mary are dating and have agreed to go to the movies. John wants to see a good murder mystery but he suspects Mary would rather see the romance flick down at the Strand, so he asks her if that's where she would like to go. Now Mary loves a good adventure film but gets the feeling that John, for whatever reason, wants to see the romance, so she agrees to go to the Strand. The situation is that they are both trying to be kind and give up their preference for the benefit of the other. The result, however, is that they both sit through a movie they don't enjoy. If they had been less *considerate* of what they *thought* the other wanted, and simply stated their own preference, they would have at least had the opportunity of dealing with the situation as it truly existed. One could then acquiesce for the *real* benefit of the other or they could compromise and enjoy both the mystery and the adventure, one this week and one the next.

Its interesting to me that we as a society need to have laws to try to insure truthtelling. We have Truth in Advertising and Truth in Lending statutes already on the books. Suppose we enforced Truth in Everyday Communications which required that everything we communicated by word or deed had to be true? We would do away with *yes men,* con men, frauds of all kinds, gossips, elevated shoes, wigs, false eyelashes, padded bras, breast implants, girdles and a lot of flirtation. We would know what we were buying in the marketplace and would know what our friends actually thought of us. More importantly, we would better know our own thoughts which motivate our actions. If we couldn't fool ourselves we would either lead more satisfying and fulfilling lives or know the reason why.

Obviously Truth in Everyday Communications wouldn't be practical to enforce, nor is it really the answer. True change is not legislated, it comes from the self. It is also encouraging to note that when we deal honestly with ourselves and with others, we are more often dealt with honestly in return.

Now that we have established more truthful communications with ourselves and others and have gotten rid of much of the emotional poison which is affecting our lives and bodies, lets see how we may become even healthier.

PRESCRIPTIONS FOR LIFE

To one degree or another we are affected by our surroundings. This does not mean just the people with whom we associate or even our physical environment, but rather how we *perceive* those people and elements. If we see birds as nasty little creatures that may deposit an ugly mess on our new car, we are going to miss out on the free-spirited soaring of Jonathan Livingston Seagull. If we see people as threatening or as tools to be utilized in the pursuit of a goal, we are going to miss the richness of friendship and the joy of sharing of experience. This would be true poverty. Fortunately perceptions may be changed and enjoyment increased.

There is a very good book on the market with the ponderous title of *The Complete Guide To Your Emotions And Your Health.* It is put out by the folks who publish Prevention Magazine and is well worth the reading. In a chapter on filling your medicine chest, for example, instead of the usual pills, capsules, ointments, suppositories and general nostrums expected to be listed, this book prescribes liberal doses of art, music, poetry and humor, with the occasional sunset, rainbow, wildflower and hug thrown in for good measure. Instead of surrounding yourself with things that say, *you must be sick, why else would I be here?,* fill your environment with elements which say, *you are alive and well, and isn't it wonderful!*

There are certain people, too, who belong in this prescription. You know the type, they appear young and alive (regardless of age) and exude a child-like innocence in the way they view things. They seem not to notice the darker side of life and give the impression of being unaware of all the unpleasantries we so often encounter. I suspect they are fully aware of life's seamier aspects, but simply choose not to concentrate on them. Instead they surround themselves with beauty and joy and are more than happy to share that environment.

You may also have noticed that such people seldom argue or debate a useless issue. They have no point to prove or argument to win, and don't need to make themselves *right* by making others *wrong*. They simply *are*. We can learn a lot from these attitudes and improve our own lives in the process.

THE SCALES OF JUSTICE

There are elements in life which need to be resolved. In our justice system we have the necessity of determining the guilt or innocence of the accused for the resolution of a case. It is easy to accept this as a *right or wrong* situation and place labels on it of *good and bad*. Crime and Punishment are inherent elements of our social order and it would be difficult to operate a large society without them. When these same value judgments are applied to everyday life, however, severe problems often arise needlessly.

In discussions we tend to choose sides and adopt viewpoints which we then feel need to be advocated and defended. Once we have locked horns in this manner it becomes very difficult to resolve the matter in other than a win or lose manner. If our *opponents* viewpoint is seen as right, doesn't that make our's wrong? And if we accept what we are saying as true, don't we then have to see their statements as false? Too often these stances lead to a rigidity of position which stunts personal learning and growth and which has very little bearing on the original issue. These usually become nothing more than trying to prove a point, establishing one's correctness to the other's incorrectness. Sure, it feels good to come out a winner, but that also necessitates the establishment of a loser.

Is it possible that there are simply other ways of looking at an issue? That there are different truths for different people?

When missionaries first encountered some of the cultures they had set out to *civilize,* many were shocked by the dress and behavior codes they found. Multilation, nudity, sexual freedom and cannibalism were completely unacceptable by the standards which the missionaries had accepted, therefore were deemed wrong and had to be changed.

By the same token, the people they met had built their own culture in a manner that worked — and was right — for themselves.

If these two groups met on neutral ground, each following the ethics of their own mores, would the bare-breasted women of the one group be judged *natural* or *offensive?* Or would it simply depend upon the point of view of the observer?

Once we can accept the idea of allowing others to be what they are without feeling the necessity of proving them wrong or changing their behavior, we have rid ourselves of yet another area of personal destruction in our own lives.

This same concept applies to the workplace and personal relationships.

DIVIDE AND CONQUER

Labor relations have long been an area of conflict between people. Labor and management have evolved into *us* and *them* positions with each side prone to saying, *look what they are doing to us!* And yet some companies have come to the understanding that they are not necessarily adversarial positions, that they're simply two sections of one operation, each of which is looking to do a job and make a living. Once this concept of *team* emerges, the result is much more satisfying and productive. Everyone can come out a winner.

Personal relationships also suffer greatly if either party has to be right to the detriment of the other. Building one's self up by knocking the other down is damaging to both parties. It allows no room for true growth or development and usually ends in bitter confrontation. Mutual respect, on the other hand, allows both parties — and the relationship as a whole — to flourish and grow. It creates two lives which are working better, instead of none. Such a relationship will find more satisfaction and enjoyment in life than one in which the bulk of the energies are spent in mutual self-destruction.

Military strategists have known for centuries that the most effective method of overcoming the enemy is to create dissention in the opposing camp. Once an army is fighting within itself it has lost sight of the real objective and has effectively given the battle away. When we learn to work *with* others rather than *against* them, our lives are not only more satisfying, but will be more effective in general.

But what does all this have to do with back problems?

ZERO DOLLARS, ZERO CENTS

I recently heard of a couple who received a closing statement bill from a creditor in the amount of $0.00. They thought it was cute and forgot about it. The next month, however, the same *bill* arrived. This went on for a period of time and was soon accompanied by a statement which warned them that their credit could be adversely affected if they didn't pay the amount indicated immediately. Letters to the company produced no relief from the threats so they finally contacted a *live* person by telephone. They were told the only way to clear the matter with the computer was to send a check for the amount stated, so they did. They sent a check in the amount of zero dollars and zero cents and soon received a *thank you* statement marked Paid In Full.

This couple's credit was now saved and they could go on about their business. But what had they gone through in the meantime? Were they able to laugh the whole matter off, as just one of those things? Or did they experience frustration, anger and even rage at the futility of trying to reason with a machine that was incapable of reasoning?

We live in an age which is becoming increasingly impersonal. At no point in recorded history has man relied so heavily on machinery and technology and institutions for *survival,* or has the human element become so unimportant. We *communicate* with computers which can only respond as they are programmed. Our entertainment consists heavily of formula programming which reinforces social game-playing and news coverage which brings us daily murder and mayhem, live and in color, to remind us of our own mortality and the fragility of our existence. We are forced into dealing with ever larger, impersonal institutions and organizations which are more interested in perpetuating their existence than in helping those they were designed to serve. We encounter ignorance and apathy everywhere and often hear the plaintive cry, *somebody should do something about it (but don't look at me).* And the list goes on.

In spite of how I'm sure all this sounds, I'm not offering social commentary as much as describing those elements which are part of the overall framework in which we live (survive), work (struggle) and play (escape), and in which there is an increasingly high incidence of back pain, chemical abuse, emotional disturbance and, occasionally, suicide. And its not surprising. We are living in an age for which we are unprepared, for which there has been little time to prepare. Our grandparents — and some of our parents — traveled by the same methods used for centuries. And yet look how we travel today. There has been more technological advancement in the last few decades than in all of previous history combined!

This can be very interesting and exciting, but it can also create anxiety, fear and stress which is often manifest in undiagnosed physical ailments and artificial dependencies. And it is not our environment which needs to be altered or changed to accomodate us, it is we who need to make ourselves more whole, more *real,* so that we may accomodate and enjoy our environment, our world. If we make our own lives work better internally we will not have the need for all the external excuses and escapes on which we so often depend.

Is this saying, then, that there is no such thing as a real back pain or injury?, that we are simply using them as escapes from a world we cannot manage?

Of course not. There are certainly real injuries and deficiencies in the back just as in any other part of the body. We have broken arms, ingrown toenails, dental carries, tumors, bladder infections and back pains. But we also have ulcers, asthma, high blood pressure, headaches and back pains, *some* of which may be reduced or eliminated completely by better management of our own lives.

So do yourself a favor and take some time to look at your life. Is it working? Examine your attitudes and beliefs, your relationships and dealings with other people. Are they what you want? What about your employment and financial conditions? Are you satisfied? Do you believe in your goals and aspirations? Whose expectations are you working to fulfill? Are the expectations for yourself and others what you really want?

Don't worry, these are very personal questions and no one needs to hear the answers except you, unless you wish to share them with someone else.

After you have gone through the above, ask yourself one more question. "Are my answers honest?" You might be surprised at what you will find and by the positive changes which may take place in your life.

Besides, what do you have to lose?

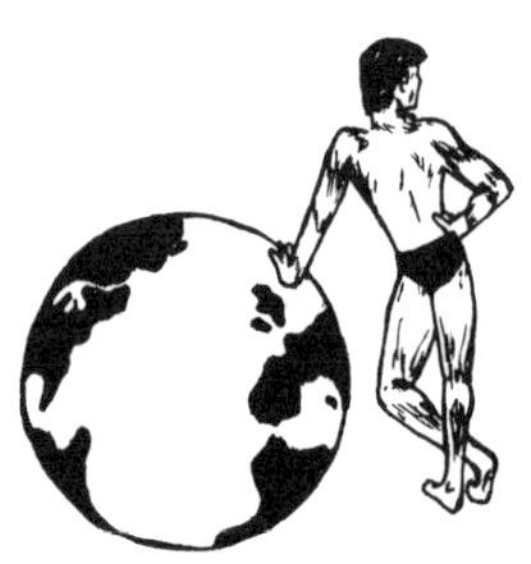

Appendix

SURVEY RESULTS

In preparing to put this book together, I was interested in seeing what the guy and gal *down the street* had to say about their experiences with back problems. So I prepared a questionaire and passed out copies to various and sundry on a word-of-mouth basis. Although the number of responses was far from overwhelming, the information received proved to be quite interesting. Many of the findings were pretty much what I was expecting, based upon my own experience, and some of the replies surprised me. While this is far from a scientific survey and is not meant to represent anything other than informal findings, it was administered as fairly as possible. The forms, for example, were not distributed through physician's or chiropractor's offices or pain clinics as that would tend to form a biased response ratio. Nor were they limited to one geographical area. Replies were received from the states of New York, California, Vermont and Maryland in order to avoid any concentration of *fad* or *clique* responses.

The survey form asked for responses only from "individuals who experience or who have experienced severe back pain on a regular or frequent basis." I didn't want to adulterate the information with reports from people who tripped while skipping rope as a child and have been fine ever since. Here, then, are the general results of that survey.

Seventy-five percent of the respondents were male, between the ages of 25 and 55. Four percent were under 25 and twenty-one percent were over 55. Over two-thirds reported three or more episodes a year on the average and over half indicated their average episode lasted from three days to a week. Where this becomes a real problem for our economy is in the amount of time lost from work. Whereas 22 percent said they don't usually miss work because of back pain, 35 percent claim they lose more than two weeks a year due to back problems. This affects not only those who lose the work, but their employers and compensation insurance carriers as well. According to Dr. Thomas P. Sculco in *Manuscript Of Rheumatology And Outpatient Orthopedic Disorders,* low back pain results in an annual loss of 1,400 work days per 1,000 workers in the United States." Estimating 100 million workers, we come up with 140 million work days lost every year in this country alone because of low back pain. That's a staggering figure! And if we add the expense of treatment to these figures, the picture becomes even costlier. According to the survey, 96 percent of those answering pay over $50 a year for treatment, 51 percent pay over $200, and for 23 percent of the responses the cost is in excess of $1,000 a year.

Interestingly enough, the types of treatment received by those individuals was evenly split at 47 percent each for medication and manipulation. The remaining 6 percent of treatment was mostly surgery, with a smattering of water therapy and acupuncture. I'll get to the results of those treatments in just a minute, but first I want to indicate what these people were going through at the time.

The questionaire asked for a response as to the severity of pain experienced during episodes of back problems. This was to be indicated on a scale of one to ten, the lower end being *discomfort* and the upper end being *sheer hell.* Eighty-three percent circled the upper end of seven through ten. While this is certainly a judgment call on the part of the individual, keep in mind that we are dealing with adults who have for the most part run the gamut of childhood illnesses, stubbed toes, toothaches and broken arms. An *eight* or *ten* response from such a person is much more meaningful than that of a seven-year old whose most traumatic experience to date has been a splinter in the finger.

As for attitudes during episodes of back pain, 79 percent indicated *long suffering,* at best, and over a third of all respondents claimed periods of gloom and depression. This substantiates my own experience and indicates some of the extended affects of back pain. Severe and repetitive bouts of pain and debility tend to erode confidence and the sense of ability, and can lead to a feeling of worthlessness. *How can I take care of my family when I can't even walk across the room?* for example. This is most unfortunate, to say the least, and brings us back to the results of treatment received during these times of great physical and emotional need.

Fortunately the majority of replies indicated an attitude of *caring* on the part of the practitioner — 56 percent for medical doctors and 69 percent for chiropractors. The rest indicated a pretty even split between *so-so* and *didn't seem to care.* Remember, this is during a time when the patient is not only in great pain, but may also be questioning their own worth. By then being seen by one of those 30-40 percent of practitioners who appear indifferent to their patient's situation only complicates the issue. None of us enjoy being served by a waitress who seems to care less whether the meal is cold or if we would like more coffee. But to see a doctor who appears indifferent to our being in the office, can be terrible.

But all the news is not bad, however. There is an interesting correlation which appears in the statistics of the survey which may prove to be beneficial in the future.

The 56 percent of medical doctors indicated as *caring,* produced 48 percent of satisfactory or better results as perceived by the patients. And the 69 percent of caring chiropractors produced 71 percent of satisfactory or better results. We can see from these numbers that the results of the treatment, as seen by the patient, follow very closely to the attitude demonstrated by the practitioner. It tells me that if *all* health-care professionals truly cared for their patient's well-being, we would see a much higher percentage of satisfying results for back pain sufferers, as well as for health care in general.

In all fairness, I would like to take just a moment to acknowledge and personally thank the *majority* of practitioners indicated in the survey. I know your patient load can sometimes be overwhelming, and we are yet another to add to your burden. But when you still take the time to make us feel as if our problem is important to you, you are adding that extra touch of caring which can make so much difference. We are aware of it and we appreciate it.

Now back to the survey. Once again, I need to point out that this survey was neither scientific or conclusive. It was, however, conducted with an eye toward fairness and was designed and distributed in a manner to help insure impartial results. It is, basically, what the man and woman down the street have found in their own experience with back problems.

I have included a copy of the actual questionaire in this chapter so you are able to see how the information was obtained and may submit your own experiences. I am interested in receiving any material which may be of help to other individuals. The form is printed back-to-back so the one leaf may be removed from the book, or you may simply provide the appropriate information on a blank sheet of paper. Thank you. (See Author's Request at the back of the book.)

Survey Results

BANNISTER PUBLICATIONS
Port Henry, N.Y. 12974

This questionnaire is to be completed only by individuals who experience
or have experienced severe back pain on a regular or frequent basis.
The results of this survey will be used in a book to be published by
Bannister Publications, and tentatively titled THE BAD BACK BOOK.
Confidentiality of name and address will be assured by checking the
appropriate box on the reverse of this form. Thank you for your co-
operation.

```
AGE GROUP:   Under 25   / /        SEX:      Male   / /
                25-40   / /                Female   / /
                40-55   / /
                55-70   / /        AVERAGE "ATTACKS"   1   / /
                over 70 / /          PER YEAR:         2   / /
                                             3 or more     / /

AFFLICTED AREA:  Lower back   / /   AVERAGE LENGTH OF   1-2 days  / /
                Center back   / /   TIME PER BOUT:      3-7 days  / /
            Upper back/neck   / /               Over a week  / /

SEVERITY OF ATTACKS (discomfort)    1 2 3 4 5 6 7 8 9 10 (sheer hell)
     on a scale of 1-10:            (Please circle one of above)

HELP SOUGHT:   Medical   / /        TREATMENT: Medication  / /
            Chiropractic / /                      Surgery  / /
            Osteopathic  / /                  Manipulation / /
                  Other  / /  __________        Other  / / ______

RESULTS OF TREATMENT:   Excellent    / /  ______________________________
                     Satisfactory    / /  ______________________________
                   Not much help     / /  ______________________________
                        No help      / /  ______________________________
                                          (list type of treatment)

ATTITUDE OF          Caring   / /   AVERAGE ANNUAL COST   Under $50  / /
PRACTITIONER:        So-so    / /     OF TREATMENT:         50-200   / /
          Didn't seem to care / /                       200-1,000   / /
                                                         over 1,000  / /

MOST PREVALENT  Slipped disc  / /   AVERAGE DAY'S WORK        0   / /
DIAGNOSIS:         Arthritis  / /   LOST ANNUALLY DUE      1-3   / /
              Strained muscle / /   TO BACK PROBLEMS:      4-7   / /
              Pulled ligament / /                        8-14   / /
            Cracked vertebrae / /                     over 14   / /
                      Other   / /  ________________

ATTITUDE OF SPOUSE/                 YOUR ATTITUDE
FAMILY:     Supportive/Cheerful / / DURING "ATTACKS":
                       Helpful  / /              Optimistic  / /
          Aggravated by demands / /          Long suffering  / /
        Doubtful of pain at all / /          Depressed/Gloomy / /
```

(Over, please)

Back Talk

Please use this space to make any general comments you wish to make,
as well as relate personal experiences which may be of interest or
assistance to the readers. (Again, confidentiality will be assured
by checking the appropriate box below.) Use additional paper if
necessary.

NAME:_________________________________TELEPHONE: (   )________________

ADDRESS: ____

          ____

I do ⧹⧸
I do not ⧹⧸   give my permission for my name/address to be used in
              the book and in its promotion and distribution.

Signed: ________________________________ Date: ______________________

Please return this form to: Bannister Publications
                             P O Box 63
                             Port Henry, NY 12974

BIBLIOGRAPHY

Cooley, Donald G. ed. *Better Homes And Gardens Family Medical Guide*. New York, New York, 1976.

Hoppenfeld, Stanley, M.D. *Physical Examination Of The Spine And Extremities*. Norwalk, Connecticut, 1976.

Iverson, Larry D. M.D. and Clawson, D. Kay, M.D. *Manual Of Acute Orthopaedic Therapeutics*, Boston, Massachusetts, 1982.

Lettvin, Maggie. *Maggie's Back Book*. Boston, Massachusetts, 1976.

McKenzie, Robin. *Treat Your Own Back*. Lower Hutt, New Zealand, 1985.

Melleby, Alexander. *The Y'S Way To A Healthy Back*. Piscataway, New Jersey, 1982.

Padus, Emrika. *The Complete Guide To Your Emotions and Your Health*. Emmaus, Pennsylvania, 1986.

Ratcliff, J.D. *I Am Joe's Body*. New York, New York, 1980.

Reilly, Brendan M., M.D. *Practical Strategies In Outpatient Medicine*. Philadelphia, Pennsylvania, 1984.

Root, Leon, M.D. and Kiernan, Thomas. *Oh, My Aching Back*. New York, New York, 1973.

Sportelli, Louis, D.C. *Introduction To Chiropractic*. 1979.

Wayne, Jerry. *The Bad Back Book*. Woodbridge, Connecticut, 1983.

Wyngaarden, James B., M.D. and Smith, Lloyd H., M.D. eds. *Cecil — Textbook Of Medicine*. Philadelphia, Pennsylvania, 1982.

The doctor of the future will give no medicine but will interest his patients in the care of the human frame, in diet and in the cause and prevention of disease.

Attributed to Thomas Edison

INDEX

AUTHOR'S REQUEST

I am very interested in hearing what you have to say about your own experiences with back pain. You may use the sample form shown in the chapter on Survey Results or, better yet, write what you have to say in a letter.

Experiences submitted may concern employment, family relations, treatments received or personal discoveries, and may be serious or humorous in nature. The information received may be used in a future publication so please indicate if you are willing for your name to be used.

Thank You.

Send all correspondence to:
J. Robert DuBois
c/o Bannister Publications
PO Box 63
Port Henry, NY 12974